S0-CJQ-075

MA

The Female Athlete

Medicine and Sport

Vol. 15

Series Editor
E. Jokl, Lexington, Ky.
Assistant Editor
M. Hebbelinck, Brussels

S. Karger · Basel · München · Paris · London · New York · Sydney

Selected Papers of the International Congress on Women and Sport,
Rome, Italy, July 4–8, 1980

The Female Athlete

A Socio-Psychological and Kinanthropometric Approach

Volume Editors
J. Borms, M. Hebbelinck (Brussels) and *A. Venerando* (Rome)

44 figures and 46 tables, 1981

S. Karger · Basel · München · Paris · London · New York · Sydney

Medicine and Sport

National Library of Medicine, Cataloging in Publication
International Congress on Women and Sport (1980: Rome, Italy)
The female athlete: a socio-psychological and kinanthropometric approach: selected
papers of the International Congress on Woman and Sport, Rome, Italy, 4–8, 1980.
Volume editors, J. Borms, M. Hebbelinck, and A. Venerando. – Basel, New York:
Karger, 1981.
(Medicine and sport; v. 15)
1. Anthropometry – congresses 2. Sports – congresses 3. Women – psychology –
congresses I. Borms, J. (Jan) II. Hebbelinck, M. (Marcel) III. Venerando, Antonio
IV. Title V. Series
W1 ME649P v.15/QT 260 I565f 1980
ISBN 3–8055–2739–X

Drug Dosage

The authors and the publishers have exerted every effort to ensure that drug selection and dosage set forth in this text are in accord with current recommendations and
practice at the time of publication. However, in view of ongoing research, changes
in government regulations, and the constant flow of information relating to drug
therapy and drug reactions, the reader is urged to check the package insert for each
drug for any change in indications and dosage and for added warnings and pre-
cautions. This is particularly important when the recommended agent is a new and/or
infrequently employed drug.

All rights reserved
No part of this publication may be translated into other languages, reproduced or
utilized in any form or by any means, electronic or mechanical, including photo-
copying, recording, microcopying, or by any information storage and retrieval system, without permission in writing from the publisher.

© Copyright 1981 by S. Karger AG, P.O. Box, CH-4009 Basel (Switzerland)
Printed in Switzerland by Tanner & Bosshardt AG, Basel
ISBN 3–8055–2739–X

617.1027
M469
v. 15

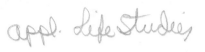

The Female Athlete

This volume contains 21 selected papers presented at the *International Congress on Women and Sport*, Rome, July 4–8, 1980. 31 further papers are published as Women and Sport. An Historical, Biological, Physiological and Sportsmedical Approach, forming vol. 14 in the series Medicine and Sport (for contents see pp. VII)

Contents

Kinanthropometry

Biomechanics

Women and Sport

An Historical, Biological, Physiological and Sportsmedical Approach

31 selected papers presented at the *International Congress on Women and Sport*, Rome, July 4–8, 1980. Published as vol. 14 in the series Medicine and Sport

Contents

Contents

Biology and Biochemistry of Exercise

Physiology of Exercise

Sportsmedical Aspects

Contents

Preface

Sport reflects values found in our everyday lives and even in our entire society. Women have been excluded from certain areas of significant participation in various aspects of living and this is also true for their involvement in sport and other physical activities. There is perhaps no domain where myths, attitudes and beliefs remain so persistent as in the world of sports. There are myths related to the female's physical and psychological masculinization, the female's monthly cycle, pregnancy, the female's physical and psychological limits of performance capacity, etc. Most of these beliefs are rooted in long sociocultural attitudes; however, their validity has not been demonstrated scientifically. Social approval is relative. It differs from era to era and from culture to culture within a given era. There are nations which actively oppose any competitive efforts for women. Other nations urge their women to enter the Olympics, while still others merely permit them to do so. However, even today some forms of competition are officially unacceptable for women as indicated by their exclusion from Olympic level competition. Perhaps an explanation for these attitudes could be found in the history of sport, colored by male orientation and domination. Such a domination resulted from cultural patterns and perceptions which determined not only who participated in sport but how the sport was to be conducted and experienced. However, today sport is seen as human activity, not just an activity more suitable for men than for women.

Women's sport is expanding rapidly, but we must realize that the situation is not entirely satisfactory. For example, if one looks at the participation either in recreational sports by women in local communities, or at the international level of sport competitions, it is clear that women do not enjoy enough equal opportunities to fully engage in sports.

In a 14-nation study of the working mother, conducted under the auspices of UNESCO and published in 1967, it was shown that women in general work longer hours and have less leisure time than men. This means that both categories of women, the working and the non-working, are at a disadvantage as compared with men. Mainly the working women have the largest disadvantage because they are still doing the major part of the household and family-raising work. However, the housewives are also disadvantaged because their labors are underestimated and most often do not follow a fixed and limited working schedule. Even if the burdens of the domestic work have been considerably lightened it is more difficult for a woman to find opportunities for participation in sport.

Myths and attitudes die hard but they do die. New attitudes are built slowly and will perhaps be accompanied by new myths. However, the world does change and the sex roles in our societies are changing too. Not only are women State Presidents, Prime Ministers or Chairpersons of Parliament, but we also have outstanding sportswomen which attract young girls and women to engage in sports. In 1960 Wilma Rudolph ran off with three gold medals in Rome. The world was shocked for several reasons. Firstly, female athletes not to mention black female athletes had never performed so outstandingly and secondly, Wilma Rudolph was accepted as a most attractive woman to grace magazines and television. Suddenly, the mass media discovered women's sport and this has been an ever-growing phenomenon featuring such great athletes as Olga Korbut and Nadia Comaneci, Nancy Green, Cornelia Enders, Billy Jean King, Chris Evert, Anne Marie Pröhl and many others. Today, girls and women are entering more and more sports, which are being added to regular athletic events. For example, women's rowing was first introduced to the Olympic Games in Montreal in 1976. Women's participation in so-called exclusive 'men's sports' such as road races, soccer, long-distance swimming and marathon running has increased more significantly than ever before.

This increased participation both in number and quality has naturally raised the question of scientific investigation and study in the area of women and sport. It is an important issue but the gap of scientific knowledge in this field is still enormous. Not only is women's involvement in the world of sport science still restricted but furthermore only a small part of the scientifically related literature deals with women's performance or compares men and women under conditions of maximum effort. There are almost no studies concerning the long-range effects of intensive conditioning programs on women. There is no overwhelming information on the physical capabilities of older women. Assessment of the female function in sport and exercise has mainly been generalized from results of investigations of male participants. Sport standards were in fact male and thus the women in sport were compared more with men than with other women.

Hence, scientific facts are needed and therefore scientific congresses can possibly help in solving these problems. Rome was the site of the 1980 *Women and Sport* Conference, which assembled nearly 500 people from many different countries.

This volume is not exclusively about differences or similarities between women and men. It is a book on women living and playing in the sports environment. This book will not give solutions to all problems, but it will identify them and attempt to give a better insight in the athletic potential of all women. This book contains only a *selected* number of papers presented in Rome, July 1980. The papers present a multi-disciplinary perspective to the issue of the female athlete and are arranged in four chapters which reflect the structure of the congress. Each part is introduced by a specialist in her or his own right on the topic selected. The book starts with papers dealing with the sociological aspects, while Dr. *D. Harris'* (University Park) paper on the implications of personality research for women in sport serves as an introduction to the sport psychology chapter. Dr. *W.D. Ross* and colleagues (Burnaby, B.C.) deal with proportionality and body composition in female olympic athletes. Their contribution serves as the introduction of the important chapter on kinanthropometry. Finally, one single paper by Dr. *D. Miller* (Seattle), selected from the biomechanical session, concludes this book.

Volume 14 of the Karger Series on Medicine and Sport *(Women and Sport)* contains selected papers from the Rome Conference dealing with historical, biological, physiological and sportmedical aspects.

The Editors are most grateful for the genuine international scientific collaboration shown by the reviewers, listed at the beginning of this book, whose expertise and professional dedication helped us significantly in this delicate task. We greatly acknowledge the efforts made by the organizing committee, the scientific and technical secretariat, the chairpersons, introducers, speakers from all countries and last but not least Karger Verlag for the production of the book. Even if a book cannot answer all questions it is hoped that its fundamental and theoretical impact will be appealing equally to women *and* men interested in the scientific assessment of women and sport and to those many practitioners who sedulously work day after day for the public acceptance and worldwide development of all sport for all women.

Brussels and Rome, January 1981.   *J. Borms*
                                                                                      M. Hebbelinck
                                                                                      A. Venerando

Reviewers

P.O. Åstrand
O. Bar-Or
G. Beunen
J. Borms
J. Broekhoff
L. Carter
A.T. Cheska
A. Dal Monte
L. Diem
B. Drinkwater
W. Duquet
D. Harris
M. Hebbelinck
H. Howald
R. Howell
J. Hueting
E. Jokl

J. Kane
J. Karlsson
H. Kemper
H. Knuttgen
P. Komi
M. Lämmer
G. Lüschen
R.C. Nelson
J. Poortmans
L. Prokop
R. Renson
W.D. Ross
S.E. Strauzenberg
B. Van Gheluwe
A. Venerando
J. Wilmore

Sociological Approach

Medicine Sport, vol. 15, pp. 1–11 (Karger, Basel 1981)

Women's Sports – The Unlikely Myth of Equality

A.T. Cheska

University of Illinois, Urbana-Champaign, Ill., USA

Introduction

This paper is about women, sports, equality or – more specifically – the lack of it. Its purposes are to demonstrate the following four propositions: (1) Women are perceived as different from men both biologically and socially, thus leading to culturally defined, specifically appropriate gender roles in varying societies of the world historically and currently. (2) Differentiated rather than equal sex status in any perceived societal context is modeled after human hierarchy. (3) Sports by their very structure are hierarchical and have chiefly functioned in the homosocial domain as models of power in industrialized or 'modern' societies. (4) Gender roles are specific over time and space; therefore, these roles can be changed. To this author the status of men and women in sports historically has been one of differentiation and inequality. However, in sports participation egalitarianism may become normative behavior in specific societies by the adoption of one or several alternatives: (a) adoption of valued male gender traits by females or vice versa in the same sports activities; (b) equal valuation of differing male and female gender traits in sports participation; (c) valuation of integrated human traits regardless of gender (androgyny). These potential alternatives are highly speculative propositions, because in the past equality has been an unlikely myth. The supportive rationale for my assumptions is not strictly based on empirically proven hypotheses, but on an historical and speculative interpretation.

Biosocial Differentiation in Gender Roles

Let us examine the first proposition, that women are perceived both biologically and socially different from men, thus leading to culturally defined gender roles for women and men in varying societies of the world. Approximately one half of the world's human population is female. The biological female's internally oriented sex organs provide the environmental receptacle for the male's sex organ. This union leads to impregnation and duplication of the couple into one sex or the other with much overlap of genetic characteristics. In all human societies it is recognized that women bear the children [*Mead*, 1949, p. 60]. Evolutionarily the birth and infant nurturance has been the female's responsibility. Historically the male was the protector and keeper of territorial boundaries. Both provided food for the group; the males hunted high protein game and the females foraged and gathered complementary foodstuffs and roots. The in- and near-camp activities of the female and the farther journeys of the male seem to have special significance in the division of labor, and from these behaviors developed further projections of socially valued gender roles [*Martin and Voorhies*, 1975]. Scholars have tried to bridge the equivalency of sex roles to that of gender roles, contending that the 'protected' female gradually became recognized as property of the male as well as his status object (there is ample evidence of this condition in animal behavior). Frequently the leap from sexual division of labor to attributions of hierarchy, power, or prestige is tacitly assumed, as if no elaboration is needed [*Parker and Parker*, 1979, p. 289]. Because gender traits are assigned symbolically, not biologically, this quantum leap is dangerous. However, here the social exchange theory can be used to account for institutionalization of asymmetrical sex-linked power and prestige in the development of human society.

Specificity of societal gender roles was first pointed out by anthropologist *Margaret Mead*. She documented ethnographically varying gender roles among primitive societies. Making the survey of competitive, cooperative, and individualistic habits among 13 cultures, *Mead* [1961] was able to identify a wide range in gender role expression. She also contrasted the gentle, cooperative, nurturant Arapesh people of New Guinea with the aggressively competitive Mundugumor living just 10 miles away. The Tuchambuli stood in contrast to both the Arapesh and Mundugumor in that the female was impersonal, skillfully competent, and dominant, while the male was dependent and aesthetically oriented [*Mead*, 1969]. She identified sex role diversity between and within societies. Today the variability of gender roles is com-

monly accepted. *Lipman-Blumen* [1976, pp. 17, 18] analyzes this differentiation in western societies: 'In relationships between the sexes, males have
had a disproportionate amount of resources under their control. They could
bargain their power, status, money, land, political influence, legal power,
and educational and occupational resources (all usually greater than wom-
en's) against women's more limited range of resources, consisting of sexu-
ality, youth, beauty, and the promise of paternity. Men also could bargain
their aggression, strength, competitiveness, and leadership capabilities
against women's domestic and clerical services. In addition, men could offer
women potential maternity, reciprocally the ultimate validation (in a sexist
world) of a woman's femininity.'

This reciprocal condition ably describes the social interaction of exchange systems. It indicates the mutual dependence of sentiment, activity,
and interaction between members of a social system [*Homans*, 1950]. This
does not imply equivalency or equality. The valuation of the above resources with which each sex has to bargain must be commonly understood
in the culture, and the uneven distribution of this valuation must also be
recognized.

Hierarchical Concept in Human Relations

This brings us to the second point, that differentiated sex status in any
perceived societal context, rather than equality, is overwhelmingly evidenced
in the pan-human concept of hierarchy. As humans have increasingly organized themselves into social groupings, whether the units were biologically
extended families or complex politico-economic nation states, the primal
human needs were linked to survival by environmental adaptive behavior.
Environment refers to the material, physical, or energy form-and-flow
aspects of man's social and physical habitat [*Adams*, 1975, p. 13]. Power is
that aspect of social relations that marks the relative control by each person
over elements of the environment of concern to the participants. Hence,
power is a socio-psychological phenomenon, whereas the control is a physical
phenomenon [*Adams*, 1975, pp. 9, 10]. He further argues: 'Power lies in the
dominance and leadership of one animal over others and in the relative
controls that the various members of the band individually or collectively
exercise over their environments. As with all living things, man's survival
depends on a continuing control over the environment. As distinct from
that of other species, the evolution of man's control has led to an ability to

endow elements of the habitat with arbitrary meanings (assigned values). The combination of the ability to invent new symbols, *culture*, and the ability to elaborate the physical skills and forms, *technology*, has provided man with an increasingly successful control, which is extremely complex and becomes more complex as culture advances' (author's italics for emphasis).

Interestingly, there is a distinction between force or physical coercion as exercise of control and power as symbolic control; for power is the set of psychosocial conditions for decision-making. However, it must be remembered that the symbolic layers of power when stripped to the core or ultimate meaning translate into the use of force for compliance. Social power can be considered the ability to get somebody else to do what you want him or her to do through your control over that person. This is a central issue in all organizational processes. The exercise of social power is one of the most important types of trigger mechanisms available to humans. The evolution of human society has been based on differential use of social power. This process has logically developed from binary differentiation, classification, and ranking or arrangement which is common to all human beings [*Adams*, 1975, p. 166]. Ranking in humans exists when there are fewer positions of valued status than persons capable of filling them. This means that members of a society enjoy differential right of access to basic resources [*Fried*, 1967, p. 52]. He implies that it is impossible to classify any society as non-ranked. The ranking of objects (or humans) involves making a judgment based on differences observed and then bestowing value. Given the differences between the sexes biologically and the classification, categories, or attributes assigned to each sex as gender roles, the inviolate result is ranking. Why specifically males have gravitated to the preferred positions of decision-making in the public domain and women in the private domain [*Rosaldo*, 1974] may be a long trial from basic application and extension of force or power upon the physical environment translated into social power. According to *Levi-Strauss* [1966] the vast majority of social organizations are asymmetrical. Binary opposition exists, but it exists hierarchically.

Hierarchical Structuring of Sports

The third assumption follows from the second. Sports by their very structure are hierarchical and have functioned chiefly in the homosocial domain as models of power in industrialized or 'modern' societies. It has taken half of this paper to get to the topic of sports; however, the foundation of differing perceived roles of women and men and the basic quality of hierarchy in human relationships had first to be established.

By definition a game is a competitive event of organized play between two or more sides with agreed-upon rules and criteria for determining the winner [*Roberts* et al., 1959, p. 597]. *Levi-Strauss* [1966, p. 32] astutely analyzes: 'Games thus appear to have a *disjunctive* effect: they end in the establishment of a difference between individual players or teams where originally there was no indication of inequality. And at the end of the game they are distinguished into winners and losers... In the case of games the symmetry is therefore preordained and it is of structural kind since it follows from the principle that rules are the same for both sides. Asymmetry is engendered: it follows inevitably from the contingent nature of events, themselves due to intention, chance or talent... Like science (though here again on both the theoretical and the practical plane) the game produces events by means of a structure; and we can therefore understand why competitive games should flourish in our industrial societies.'

Games provide excellent models of competitive striving for hierarchy or control. *Gruneau* [1975, p. 129] states it well, '...hierarchy, as a concept, is a cornerstone of the sporting ethos. Any emphasis or outcome wherein winning is at all valued is a basic statement of a distributive relationship. The winner presumably shows his or her excellence.' The traits of strength, aggression, competitiveness, and leadership capabilities can be played, practiced, and displayed in an athletic arena as an exercise of symbolic power where strategy, chance and skill as merit make a difference. The events can be repeated with potential success always attracting and tantalizing the participants. This repetition is not often possible in the world's social power interactions. It is intriguing to speculate upon the origin of power as ultimately being force or physical coersion.

This playground of power along with the need for aggregation hold powerful motivating ingredients for homosocial exchange. *Metheny* [1965] stated that the Olympic sports may well symbolize man's conception of himself as a consequential force within the grand design of the universe, as well as each man's conception of his own ability to perform those functions that identify him as a man among men. The homosocial view of gender roles suggests that men are attracted to, stimulated by, and interested in other men [*Lipman-Blumen*, 1976]. The sports situation allows men to practice their gender roles with each other [*Maccoby and Jacklin*, 1974]. *Tiger*

[1970] extensively documented this male 'bonding' phenomenon as revealed in sports, secret societies' initiation rites, war and so on. He showed how males 'court' other males and validate their maleness through interaction, often of an aggressive, even violent nature. *Lipman-Blumen* [1976] suggests that men identify with and seek help from other men because individuals identify with other individuals who they perceive to be controllers of resources in any given situation. The competitive use of physical prowess, strength, and aggression in seeking and achieving power-oriented rewards inherently carries the attribute of hierarchy. Kinetic games and sports, as models of symbolic control, reinforce status in the homosocial arena where males interact with other males. The meta-messages of sports participation include compatible aggregation, consensually determined means and goals, and participatory ordering. Historically women have been excluded as inappropriate and ineffective game contenders, whose presence was allowed in supportive service roles and as display commodities within these social power transactions.

In past eras, games served concurrently both as cultic expressions and recreative enjoyment [*Crawley*, 1913; *Culin*, 1907; *Cushing*, 1883; *Damm*, 1970; *Gini*, 1939; *Henderson*, 1947; *Massingham*, 1929; *Simri*, 1968]. Games in which males competed almost exclusively were self-testing bouts, contests or mass participation. Structurally the game consisted of assigned sides, few procedural operations, generalized interchangeable roles and responsibilities and, in sacred rites, frequently predetermined outcomes. The ritual game through iconic symbols (acts, words, or things) provided models of the power process. The ritual message condensed the varying power experiences of life and their meanings within a particular society into an objective vehicle which was understood and shared by individuals on a personal, subjective level. The ritual served to filter, solidify, unify, imagize, and legitimize the power hierarchy in interpersonal relations [*Cheska*, 1979, p. 51]. As sacred or profane ritual enactments, they both are symbolic messages of hierarchical power, the sacred representing the super-human and the profane representing the superb human [*Cheska*, 1979, p. 68]. Desacralizing games to sports has shifted the metaphor from the imitative symbol of ascribed godly power to that of achieving human power. Ritually the concept of games was one of ascription; recreationally it was one of competitive achievement; therefore, both models of power were available for males. Evolutionarily sport is an industrial age game phenomenon with more complex, differentiated roles, skills and procedures, and uncertain outcomes when compared to earlier periods. Until recently sport as power symbol has been perceived as the homosocial domain, recognizing control through attributes of competitiveness, strength, and prowess. These gender traits which are identified as masculine are also traits attributed to a successful human in western cultures [*Broverman* et al., 1975].

With few exceptions, women's past kinetic participation in games and sports has been delegated to expressive activities stressing agile body manipulation, e.g. dance or acrobatics, or light object manipulation, e.g. ball-tossing [*Abdou*, 1961; *Klafs and Lyon*, 1975; *Metheny*, 1965]. These activities carried symbolic cultic communication with religious connotations. The stress of expressiveness or quality of internally perfected performance in women's activities carried the ritualistic concept of processual excellence, modeling ascribed godly power, not that of achieving human power. These qualitative activities were seldom equated in type, style, or execution with the male games and sports which had quantified winners. However, since the modern industrialized technology has more and more included the female as worker (note women in the public market place), they have increasingly usurped the games and sports domain of the male. Competition has not be extensively with the male, but in paralleling activities. *Sutton-Smith and Rosenberg* [1961] found that girls in the United States over the past 100 years have been playing more games and sports classified as boys' activities, while boys have been narrowing their games repertoire. This has been reaffirmed by *Lever* [1976], *Sutton-Smith* [1979], *Kleiber* [1980], and *Cheska* [in press, b]. Also in the United States accelerated participation of girls and women in formal competitive sports programs has been implemented by Title IX in public schools and universities. This seems to imply the adoption by females of the kinetic male model in seeking and achieving power-oriented rewards. The logic here appears to be homologous, for if the 'same' activities are participated in by females as well as males, then the same gender traits are developed and expressed and the same results occur [*Groos*, 1901, p. 340].

Changing Gender Roles

This observation brings us to the fourth assumption of this paper. Gender roles are specific over time and space; therefore, they can be changed. The progressive logic of this paper has attempted to indicate that change over time and space is inevitable; however, there seem to be universals within which change evolves. One is the biologically differing body plans of the two sexes; the second is the evolving from binary opposition categorization to hierarchical status in social groupings. My suggestion is in sports participation that egalitarianism may become normative behavior in specific societies by the adoption of one of several alternatives. One alternative is the adoption of male gender traits by females (or vice versa) in the same sports activities. Evidence points to females in United States who participate in intercollegiate competitive sports displaying male gender traits as assertiveness, aggressiveness, competitiveness, mastery of the physical environment [*Balazs*, 1975; *Gerber*, 1974; *Harris*, 1973; *Kane*, 1972; *King and Chi*, 1979; *Kingsley* et al., 1977; *Rohrbaugh*, 1979]. The second suggestion is the equal valuation of differing male and of differing female gender traits in sports participation. This would be a double standard of value or excellence. In gymnastics competition males and female free exercise routine excellence is judged by differing criteria. Women's performance consists of approximately 60% agile, rhythmic dance exercises in which synchronized continuity, elegance, and grace are positive attributes. Strong tumbling activities may be performed, but they are to appear effortless. Men's performances consist of approximately 85% continuous strong tumbling of high degrees of difficulty and danger. About 15% is based on transitional corner moves between tumbling activities [*Leo*, 1980]. The third proposal suggests valuing of integrated human traits (androgyny) rather than those assigned to gender. Among the markers in the past, gender roles have served to distinguish specialization in most aspects of social organization, cutting wholistically across economic, religious, political, and leisure activities. However, as organizational complexity increased over time, the modes of sociospecialization also increased [*Martin and Voorhies*, 1975]. Large scale, industrialized societies, more than smaller, less differentiated societies, need increasingly to identify and use more specifically their available talent in all groupings. To adequately fulfill these diverse skill requirements, a reevaluation of poorly utilized or unused talent is demanded. Gender roles as inhibitors seem remarkably dysfunctional in complex societies and need revision.

In sports performance, research effort has gone into showing that well-conditioned male and female bodies are much more similar in lean body mass and cardiovascular performance than previous researchers assumed [*Burke*, 1977; *Drinkwater*, 1973]. These studies indirectly point to increasing equality of performance potential. However, because gender roles are assigned symbolically, not biologically, performance equality may not be relevant [*Chafetz*, 1974]. Within the world view of a people, social organization as a structure of intergroup relations becomes an identifying codification by fixing and labeling differences and values. These categories of mental organization provide a dialectic methodology for managing and ordering experiences of existence [*Cheska*, in press, a]. The socially determined perception of roles may reinforce differential valuing of sensory-motor performance as well as cognitive production. This phenomenon is noted in judging of the relative quality and worth of process and product by each sex. For example, if an intercollegiate basketball game score of 41–40 is announced by a television sportscaster without identifying the score as the men's team or the women's team, the listeners interpret the result as a close contest. When told it was the girls' team score, the listeners tend to further attribute the low score to poor playing skills; while, if told this is the males' team score, the low score is further attributed to a tight defensive game. To alleviate this bias, *Duquin* [1978] has proposed the changing of the sex-typed to the sex-natural perception of sport.

A given in culture is change, and as such, gender roles are changing; and these changes are being reflected in sports. However, it is my contention that the present women's sports participation is really a readjustment of the social power hierarchy. Given the basic social relationships of humans, equality is merely a point in passing from one dominance status to another. The fluctuations within hierarchy are historically validated. The changing of the socio-politico-economic value structure by varying groups has been termed 'his-story'. The current and future trend and potential based on societal's perception may lead to social status and value dominance of the female. However, the basic principle of hierarchy in social relations will provide a framework within which change occurs and within which change will be affirmed.

References

Abdou, K.S.: Sports and games in ancient Egypt; PhD Diss., Bloomington (1961).

Adams, R.N.: Energy and structure: a theory of social power (University of Texas, Austin 1975).

Balazs, E.: In quest of excellence (Hoctor Products for Education, Waldwick 1975).

Broverman, I.K.; Vogel, S.R.; Broverman, D.M.; Clarkson, F.E.; Rosenkrantz, P.S.: Sex-role stereotypes: a current appraisal; in Lasky Humanness: an exploration into the mythologies about women and men, pp. 29–48 (MSS Information Corporation, New York 1975).

Burke, E.J.: Physiological effects of similar training programs in males and females. Res. Q. *48:* 510–517 (1977).

Chafetz, J.S.: Masculine, feminine or human? (Peacock Publishing, Itasca 1974).

Cheska, A.T.: Sport spectacular: a ritual model of power. Rev. Sport Sociol. *14:* 51–72 (1979).

Cheska, A.T.: The ritual games as mediation structure in the Pueblo world view (in press, a).

Cheska, A.T.: Native American youth sports' choices and game attraction factors (in press, b).

Crawley, A.E.: The book of the ball (Methuen, London 1913).

Culin, S.: Games of North American Indians. 24th Annu. Rep. to the Bureau of American Ethnology (Government Printing Office, Washington 1907).

Cushing, F.H.: My adventures in Zuni, vol. III. Century Illus. mon. Mag. *16:* 28–47 (1883).

Damm, H.: The so-called sport activities of primitive people: a contribution towards the genesis of sport; in Lüschen, The cross-cultural analysis of sport and games, pp. 52–69 (Stipes Publishing, Champaign 1970).

Drinkwater, B.L.: Physiological responses of women to exercise; in Wilmore, Exercise and sport sciences reviews (Academic Press, New York 1973).

Duquin, M.E.: The androgynous advantage; in Oglesby, Women and sport from myth to reality, pp. 89–106 (Lea & Febiger, Philadelphia 1978).

Fried, M. H.: The evolution of political society (Random House, New York 1967).

Gerber, E.; Felshin, J.; Berlin, P.; Wyrick, W.: The American women in sport (Addison-Wesley, Reading 1974).

Gini, C.: Rural ritual games in Libya (berber baseball and shinny). Rural Sociol. *4:* 282–298 (1939).

Gross, K.: The play of man (translated by Elizabeth L. Baldwin from German) (Appleton, New York 1901).

Gruneau, R.S.: Sport, social differentiation, and social inequality; in Ball, Loy, Sport and social order, pp. 117–184 (Addison-Wesley, Reading 1975).

Harris, D.V.: DGWS research reports: women in sports (National Education Association, Washington 1973).

Henderson, R.W.: Ball, bat and bishop. New York: (Rockport Press, 1947; reprint by Gale Research Company, Detroit 1974).

Homans, G.C.: The human group (Harcourt, Brace, New York 1950).

Kane, J.E.: Motivation and performance; in Harris, Women and sport. A National Research Conf., pp. 141–155 (Pennsylvania State University, University Park 1972).

King, J.P.; Chi, P.S.K.: Social structure, sex-roles, and personality: comparisons of male/female athletes/nonathletes; in Goldstein, Sports, games and play: social and psychological viewpoints, pp. 115–148 (Lawrence Erlbaum Associates, Hillsdale 1979).

Kingsley, J.L.; Brown, F.L.; Seibert, M.E.: Social acceptance of female athletes by college women. Res. Q. *48:* 727–733 (1977).

Klafs, C.E.; Lyon, M.J.: The female athlete: conditioning, competition, and culture. (Mosby, St. Louis 1973).

Kleiber, D.A.: The leisure experience of males and females: a context for androgynous behavior; unpublished paper, Urbana-Champaign (1980).

Leo, J.: Personal communication, May 29, Urbana-Champaign (1980).

Lever, J.: Sex differences in the games children play. Social Probl. *23:* 478–487 (1976).

Levi-Strauss, C.: The savage mind (University of Chicago Press, Chicago 1966).

Lipman-Blumen, J.: Towards a homosocial theory of sex roles: an explanation of the sex segregation of social institutions. 2. Signs. J. Women Culture Society *1:* 15–31 (1976).

Maccoby, E.E.; Jacklin, C.N.: The psychology of sex differences (Stanford University Press, Stanford 1974).

Martin, M.K.; Voorhies, B.: Female of the species (Columbia University Press, New York 1975).

Massingham, H.J.: Heritage of man (Cape, London 1929).

Mead, M.: Male and female (Dell Publishing, New York 1949).

Mead, M.: Cooperation and competition among primitive peoples (originally published 1937; Beacon Press, Boston 1961).

Mead, M.: Sex and temperament in three primitive societies (originally published 1937; Dell Publishing, New York 1969).

Metheny, E.: Connotations of movement in sport and dance (Wm. C. Brown, Dubuque 1965).

Parker, S.; Parker, H.: The myth of male superiority: rise and demise. Am. Anthrop. *81:* 289–309 (1979).

Roberts, J.M.; Arth, M.J.; Bush, R.R.: Games in culture. Am. Anthrop. *61:* 597–605 (1959).

Rohrbaugh, J.B.: Femininity on the line. Psychol. Today *13:* 30–42 (1979).

Rosaldo, M.Z.: Women, culture and society: a theoretical overview; in Rosaldo, Lamphere, Woman, Culture and Society; pp. 17–42 (Stanford University Press, Stanford 1974).

Simri, U.: The religious and magical function of ball games in various cultures; in Simri, Proc. 1st Int. Seminar on the History of Physical Education and Sport, pp. 2–1 to 2–20 (Wingate Institute, Netanya 1968).

Sutton-Smith, B.: The play of girls; in Kapp, Kirkpatrick, Becoming female: perspectives on development, pp. 229–257 (Plenum Publishing, New York 1979).

Sutton-Smith, B.; Rosenberg, B.G.: Sixty years of historical change in the game preferences of American children. J. Am. Folklore *74:* 17–46 (1961).

Tiger, L.: Men in groups (Random House, New York 1970).

Dr. A.T. Cheska, University of Illinois, Urbana-Champaign, IL 61801-3895 (USA)

Medicine Sport, vol. 15, pp. 12–29 (Karger, Basel 1981)

Attitudes to Women in Sport
Preface towards a Sociological Theory

E.A.E. Ferris

London, England

The Orthodox View

The orthodox view about women in sport is that, when compared with males, females have always held, and will always continue to hold, an inferior position in sporting achievement. The reasons given to support this view of female inferiority in sporting performance is that there are inherent biological factors that necessarily limit female performance potential. These factors include such things as height, body composition, muscle mass and endurance, and cardiovascular endurance capacity which, when grouped together, are taken to constitute biological differences between the sexes. In general, men are taller, heavier, stronger, have larger hearts and lungs and more muscle mass than women. Women, by contrast, are, on average, smaller, weaker, lighter and fatter than men. Sport, for the most part, requires strength, power, speed and endurance – capacities with which men are, in principle, better equipped.

At first sight, if one is stating a generalization then the orthodox view appears to be right because the beliefs supporting the view appear to be true – prima facie at any rate. In addition, these biological factors are believed to be inherent as they have their origins in genetic and hormonal endowments: hence, so the argument goes, they are fixed and immutable. And lastly, their immutability confers on the 'orthodox view' the stamp of inevitability. Furthermore, the social conditions and the male/female roles in sport that have been the natural result of this 'orthodox view', are also said to be justified and inevitable.

Sport, besides requiring certain physical attributes on the part of the athlete, also requires specific psychological characteristics. To be able to take part in sporting activity an athlete needs to manifest competitiveness, self-assertion, independence, controlled aggression, the will to win and the ability to dominate his or her opponent. These attributes are the same as those that are designated stereotypically 'masculine' – that is, normal, desirable and appropriate in the male. And, by contrast, abnormal, undesirable and inappropriate in the female.

Women possessing these traits are considered to be deviant. The typical womanly temperament includes being passive, non-competitive, submissive, nurturing and non-achievement orientated. These characteristics are supposed to be possessed *naturally* only by women, and have been designated feminine as a result. Men manifesting such traits are deemed to be out of the range of the normal male, and indeed are treated derogatorily, just as so-called 'masculine' women are treated as social misfits.

The 'biological argument' concerning the different social roles of men and women claims that psychological sex differences have genetic and hormonal origins and so, like physical sex differences, they too are fixed and immutable. Sport requires both the physical and the psychological make-up that we regard as masculine, and that males only are believed to possess by virtue of inherent biological factors which govern the development of these traits. It is no wonder that sport has always been a male domain. Whilst women do trespass on men's sporting territory, they are, at best, simply tolerated.

Attempts to Eliminate Inequalities Inherent in 'Orthodox View'
not Successful

Since the inception of the women's liberation movement in the late 1960s, trends towards equality for men and women have developed. We have entered an era in which many Western countries have outlawed sexual discrimination, and have even introduced legislation to ensure equality of opportunity between the sexes in education, jobs, etc.

Sport has followed suit to some extent in these trends towards greater participation by women. In the Olympic Games in Rome in 1960, women competed in only eight sports. In Moscow this year (1980), women will compete in 14 of the 21 sports. But notwithstanding legislation to create the environment for women's emancipation, we have seen what amounts to token gestures rather than a social revolution in terms of equality of opportunity.

In sport, as well, the trend towards greater participation of women has only paid lip-service to real equality. Women were still not allowed to run further than 1,500 m in the Olympic Games in Moscow (1980), even though all the criteria for inclusion of longer events for women right up to the marathon (26 miles 385 yards) had been satisfied. The reason given by the International Olympic Committee (IOC) for its rejection of the application by the International Amateur Athletic Federation for the inclusion of a 3,000 m race for women was that 'it is a little too strenuous'[1]. But built in to the notion of lip-service to equality is the ingrained view that women's inferiority still exists. Otherwise, why should women cyclists who have been eligible for competing in the Olympic Games for decades, have had their application rejected first of all by their own male-dominated federation, and then by the IOC? And why should the international Judo Federation be having such a difficult time trying to get women's judo included in the Olympics? And why should an 11-year-old girl, Teresa Bennett, who was picked on merit to play on a boy's soccer team, be prevented from doing so by the English Football Association?

Well-meaning, morally aware people may be deeply committed to the justice of equality of opportunity between the sexes. But whilst the deeply embedded conviction is still implicitly held that women are unsuited to particular activities because of biological limitations, any progress towards real equality will be slow and ineffectual. Why? Because the view is so all-pervading that it lies below the conscious level at which critical discussion can take place. This is particularly true in the field of sporting endeavour. It is this tension between the desire to be egalitarian on the one hand, and our holding the 'orthodox view', however subliminally and even non-propositionally, on the other, that prevents real progress.

The 'orthodox view' has been further reinforced by comparisons of performance standards in men and women in various events. Performances by women in track and field events are significantly inferior to those of men, and much has been written to explain why this is so and, so it is asserted, always will be so [*Lietzke*, 1954; *Lloyd*, 1966].

The Orthodox View Refuted

Evidence from Performance
I wish to question the 'orthodox view' of women's sporting inferiority. I am interested in demonstrating that people's actual abilities far outstrip

---

[1] It was decided by the IOC in 1980 that in the Olimpic Games to be held in Los Angeles in 1984, women will compete in the 3000 m track and in the marathon.

what, at any moment, they think they are capable of, and that they tend to conform in their behaviour and achievements to accepted and *acceptable* standards and values based on current views and expectations. I am suspicious of the ascription of inherent, biologically determined constraints limiting sporting performance in human beings. Records are always being broken and barriers overcome in the field of sporting endeavour that were hitherto considered to be impossible due, it was thought, to limitations in human ability; the 4-min mile, the 7-ft high-jump, climbing Everest, and many many more besides.

These barriers and records have always been overcome and set by men. But, in the last two decades, as women have invaded the arena of sporting endeavour, they too have set new world standards. Let us look at some of the evidence.

The two-way Channel record swim is held by a woman, Cynthia Nicholas, of Canada. Another woman, Penny Lee Dean (USA), holds the England to France record. Women have climbed Everest. Until a few weeks ago, Dame Naomi James (NZ) held the round-the-world, solo-sailor record. Again, Ann Sayer holds the record for the gruelling, 7-day Three Peaks Walk. Betty Cook won the World Powerboat Title in 1979. Also last year, a woman jockey, Ann Ferris (no relation), won the Irish Hurdles steeplechase and yet another, Bev Francis of Australia, set a women's world record in a *men's* middleweight weightlifting competition beating all the men in the event along the way. In cycling, Beryl Burton of Great Britain, many time holder of the world title, riding in a 12-h event, created a new competition record and covered 277 miles, two more than her closest male rival. Another enduring female, Gail Roy, set a new high altitude ballooning record in 1979 without the aid of oxygen. These are but a few examples. So we see that women have not only begun to perform physical feats of which they were believed to be 'biologically' incapable, but in certain events, they have even excelled over men. The orthodox view is already showing weaknesses.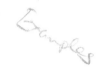

Gap between Women's Records and Men's Records Closing

For further evidence to support our argument that the 'orthodox view' is wrong, let us examine empirical data in the form of male and female world record performances, and discover the trends contained therein. Analyses of actual performances in sporting events involving strenuous exertion, such as swimming and running, have revealed that when compared with the men's records, the women's performances are improving at a faster rate at almost

Table I. World records for the marathon (in hours, min and sec) for men and women and their percentage difference[1], 1963–1979

Year	Men	Women	Difference, %
1963	2:15:15.8	3:37:07	37.21
1963	2:14:43.0		37.93
1964	2:13:55.0	3:27:45	35.43
1964	2:12:11.2		36.28
1965	2:12:00.0	3:19:33	33.96
1967	2:09:36.4	3:15:22.8	33.70
1967		3:07:26.2	30.94
1969	2:08:33.3		31.44
1970		3:02:53	29.62
1971		3:01:42	29.25
1971		3:00:35	28.88
1971		2:56:30	27.24
1971		2:55:22	26.69
1971		2:49:40	24.31
1973		2:46:36	22.85
1974		2:46:24	22.67
1974		2:43:54.5	21.57
1975		2:42:24	20.84
1975		2:40:15.8	19.74
1975		2:38:19	18.83
1977		2:35:15.4	17.18
1977		2:34:47.5	17.00
1978		2:32:29.8	15.72
1979		2:27:33	12.80
1980		2:25:40	11.70

[1] Expressed as a percentage of the men's world record.

all distances [*Dyer*, 1976, 1977; *Ferris*, 1977, 1979]. *Dyer* [1977] made statistical analyses of male and female world records in track, swimming and cycling between 1948 and 1976, and he states that: 'The overall performance by females in each of these three sports has significantly improved relative to male performance during the years in question.' With respect to track events (100, 200, 800, 4 × 100 and 4 × 200 m) *Dyer* [1977] calculated the mean percentage difference between male and female world track athletics records. The mean percentage difference in these events diminished from 16.85% in 1948, to 10.46% in 1976. This steady decline in the difference between the sexes is reflected in the world records of all the track events. In some cases,

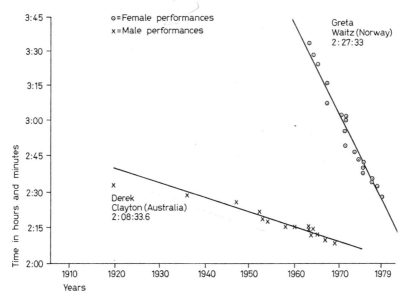

Fig. 1. Trends in improvement in world best performances of men and women in the marathon.

the differences have declined by more than half. For instance, in the 800 m the percentage difference was 20.33% in 1948, and 9.98% in 1976.

Interestingly, *Dyer* [1977] notes that: 'The performance differential for athletic events... appears to be declining more rapidly in recent years as the longer events are introduced.' In other words, it is in the longer-distance events, in which women have been competing for the least time, that the greatest decline in the percentage difference between the male and female records is occurring.

The marathon is the outstanding example of this trend (table I). In the 11 years between 1969 and 1980, the percentage difference between the male and female world best times declined by nearly two-thirds from 31.44 to 1.70%. The men's record held by Derek Clayton of Australia has remained unchanged during this period at 2:08:33.3, whilst the women's record has decreased by marathon more than 40 min (21%). Figure 1 shows the male and female world records in the marathon. It illustrates that the rate of improvement in the women's performance far exceeds that of the men. (As the numbers of women running marathons increases and the mileage covered by them in training also increases, we may expect this rate of improvement in female standards to continue or even to accelerate.)

Table II. World records (in min and sec) for women in freestyle swimming events in 1960 and 1979 and the year the men's world record first exceeds the women's

Event	Women's records 1960	Year men's record first exceeds women's 1960 record	Women's records 1979	Year men's record first exceeds women's 1979 record
100 m	1:00.2	1922	55.41	1956
200 m	2:11.6	1927	1:58.23	1964
400 m	4:44.5	1934	4:06.28	1969
800 m	9:55.6	1934	8:24.62	1972
1,500 m	19:23.6	1927	16:04.49	1969

In freestyle swimming in 1960, women were lagging between 26 and 38 years behind the men in performance levels (table II) with an average lag time of 32 years. By 1979, the lag was reduced to between 23 and 7 years, with an average of 13 years. Mark Spitz' world record for the 400-m freestyle, set in 1968, would today be beaten by the 17-year-old Australian woman, Tracey Wickham. Again, three American teenage girls, Cynthia Woodhead, Kim Lineham and Mary Meagher, set world records last year (1979) in the 200-m freestyle, the 1,500-m freestyle, and the 200-m butterfly respectively that would have won each of them a gold medal in these men's events at the 1968 Olympic Games. Table III shows the percentage difference between male and female world records in freestyle swimming events, 1936–1979, and here too the trend is clearly towards women closing the gap with men in performance levels. In addition, as in running, it is in the longer events that the performance differential is the smallest. According to *Dyer* [1976] the relative difference between the sexes in running and swimming is likely to go on declining and may, eventually, disappear completely. He calculated that the linear regressions of the mean differences in male and female performances between 1948 and 1976 predict equality between the sexes in cycling, swimming and running within 50 years. He further states that the predictions that emerge from a systematic analysis of the data, such as he has made, 'suggest that assumptions concerning the effects of physical and physiological differences between males and females will need to be reconsidered, and that, in the past, it was social and psychological factors which held back female sporting performance as much as physiological factors' [*Dyer*, 1977].

Table III. Percentage difference[1] between male and female world records in freestyle swimming 1936–1979

Event	Difference between world records in			
	1936	1956	1966	1979
100 m	12.69	10.64	10.19	10.68
200 m	12.45	10.91	10.96	7.14
400 m	11.81	7.14	8.60	6.36
800 m	11.00	11.92	8.58	5.36
1,500 m	30.82	12.26	8.35	6.02
Mean difference all events	15.75	10.57	9.34	7.11

[1] Expressed as a percentage of the male world record time for the event.

Physiological Characteristics Relevant to Sporting Activity Re-examined

I want now to discuss various studies of the physiological characteristics of the sexes and how these relate to their sporting abilities.

The popular belief is that females suffer from an inadequate and inefficient cardiovascular capacity to respond to vigorous exercise and that therefore they should be protected from exposure to it. In fact studies show that females respond to exercise and to strenuous training in much the same way as do men [*Kilbom*, 1971; *Roskamm*, 1967; *Cunningham and Hill*, 1975; *Edwards*, 1974; *Flint* et al., 1974].

In a review article, *Wilmore* [1979] synthesized results from previous studies on both sexes in the areas of body composition and physique, muscle fibre characteristics, strength and cardiovascular endurance capacity. He discovered that whilst there are rather substantial differences between the *average* female and the *average* male in almost all aspects of physical and physiological performance beyond the age of 10–12 years, recent studies on highly trained female athletes suggest that the female is not much different from her highly trained male counterpart beyond puberty, particularly when comparisons are made between male and female athletes who are competing in the same event or sport [*Burke and Brush*, 1979]. According to *Wilmore* [1979], it appears that the *average* values for men and women have been obtained from studies that compared relatively active males with relatively sedentary females, and that what appear to be dramatic biological differences between the sexes in physical attributes and physiological functioning in response to exercise are more related to a difference in life style. Women assume a much more sedentary existence owing to the cultural and social restrictions placed upon them after puberty. It is well-known that a substantial reduction in physical activity results in a deterioration in the basic physiological components of physical fitness; strength, cardiovascular endurance and muscular endurance all diminish and body fat accumulates. It is exactly in these features that the average female differs from the average male. However, comparisons of highly trained male and female athletes revealed more similarities than differences in these physiological and physical parameters.

With respect to strength, the traditional view is that women are considerably weaker than men. Studies have shown that whilst this is true in the upper part of the body, the lower body strength in females, in particular that in the legs, when expressed relative to body weight, is only slightly less than that in males, and when expressed relative to lean body weight, females are actually stronger in the legs than males [Wilmore, 1974]. It was also found that with a programme of progressive weight training, females can substantially increase their strength. Wilmore [1974] found that in a relatively short 10-week programme a group of young non-athletic women improved their strength by 30–50%. These relative gains were similar to those exhibited by a group of non-athletic young men on an identical programme. The only difference was that in the women practically no muscular hypertrophy occurred, whereas in the men the increase in muscle bulk was substantially greater.

In a study on seven track-and-field women athletes undergoing a strenuous 6-month training programme which included weight training with near maximal resistance exercises, increases in upper body (bench press) strength of 15–44%, and in lower body (half-squat) strength of 16–53% were obtained. The absolute values in terms of pounds lifted were considerably greater than the average, untrained male of similar age can achieve [Brown and Wilmore, 1974].

With respect to body composition, the average female is considerably fatter than the average male of the same age (25 versus 15% fat). Studies on female athletes by Wilmore et al. [1977] however have revealed that long-distance runners have relative body fats that are considerably lower than the average female and the average male. In fact, several of these women distance runners are competing for leanness with their male long-distance counterparts, with relative body fat values of less than 10%.

Costill et al. [1970] reported an average value of 7.5% fat for 114 male competitors in the 1968 United States Olympic marathon trial. Two of *Wilmore's* elite women distance runners had values of approximately 6%.

With respect to endurance capacity measured as the maximal oxygen uptake ($VO_{2\,max.}$), studies of young untrained subjects reveal what appears to be a substantial sex difference in aerobic power with female capacity only 70–75% of that in the male [*Drinkwater*, 1973]. In young trained subjects, however, this difference almost totally disappears. In a study of young elite female distance runners the values obtained for $VO_{2\,max.}$ were equivalent to those obtained for males of similar age and performance capacity [*Burke and Brush*, 1979]. The mean $VO_{2\,max}$ of 63.24 ml/kg · min^{-1} was among the highest ever recorded for a group of women. *Wilmore and Brown* [1974] obtained a mean $VO_{2\,max}$ value of 67.4 ml/kg · min^{-1} for the three best athletes of a group of mature female long-distance runners, which compares very equitably with the value of 69.7 ml/kg · min^{-1} reported for Derek Clayton, the holder of the world's best marathon performance with a time of 2:08:33 [*Costill* et al., 1971].

In addition, comparisons have been made between the thermoregulatory function in males and females, performing strenuous exercise in hot environments. *Wells* [1977] postulates that women are more efficient regulators of their body temperatures because females rely to a greater degree on cardiovascular measures of thermoregulation than on evaporative heat loss. *Morimoto* et al. [1967] found that women were apparently able to achieve thermoregulation in an environment with 80% humidity with a lower sweat rate than the men. *Weinman* et al. [1967] reported that for work in a moist heat, men had significantly higher sweat rates, whilst the women had smaller increases in heart rate and rectal temperature. Studies on acclimatization achieved by repeated exposures to work in the heat showed that in men, the extra heat is dissipated by increased body sweating. In women, however, despite the usual evidence of acclimatization, several investigators [*Weinman* et al., 1967; *Hertig* et al., 1963] have observed only a slight increase in sweat rate. According to *Wells* [1977], 'these studies suggest that women may be more efficient regulators of body temperature since they achieve the same acclimatization results with the loss of less water'. It has even been claimed by *Wyndham* et al. [1965], that 'The male... is a prolific, wasteful sweater, whereas the female adjusts her sweat rate to the required heat loss.'

More recently, *Wells and Paolone* undertook to study sex differences in *physically fit* subjects in response to exercise under heat stress conditions. From their results, they came to the same conclusions, namely that: 'Evaporative cooling for the men was not as effective in meeting the requirements of exercising in the heat' [*Wells*, 1977]. It was also demonstrated in both this and the *Weinman* et al. [1967] study that males show an increased metabolic cost of exercise in the heat when compared with females. These various results led *Wells* [1977] to suggest that 'a greater cardiovascular component of thermoregulation existed in women... (which) may be less costly than increased dependence on evaporative heat loss' as occurs in men.

These observations are particularly relevant with respect to marathon running. It is well-documented that two of the potentially more dangerous physiological aspects of marathon running are the rise in core body temperature and the loss of fluid from sweating. As physically fit women sweat less and have smaller rises in rectal temperature when strenuously exercising, in addition to having a lower metabolic cost of exercise in hot conditions, we can reasonably assume that women may be better suited physiologically to long-distance running than men. This hypothesis is supported by the observation that most women do not finish marathons in the extremely exhausted, collapsed condition most men do that is typical of the heat stress state.

To summarize, the following evidence exists: (1) in many sporting events, women have performed as well as, and on occasions better than their male counterparts; (2) in running and swimming, female performances are improving at a faster rate than male performances, showing a trend in top world achievements towards equality between the sexes in the very near future; (3) physiological research reveals that highly trained female athletes are very similar in their capacities with respect to exercise to their highly trained male counterparts.

Hence, we can reasonably reach the following conclusions: firstly the evidence put forward above severely undermines the 'orthodox view' of women's inherent sporting inferiority. The argument given to support the 'orthodox view' is that inherent biological factors *necessarily* limit a female's sporting achievement *because they are fixed and immutable*. The evidence presented in this paper suggests that the biological factors are not fixed and immutable; when a female becomes a highly trained athlete, the biological factors as manifest in physiological functioning and physical characteristics change, with the result that such women have similar capacities in these respects to equivalently trained men.

Secondly, we can reasonably conclude that there are actually good reasons for anticipating that in certain endurance events, female performance *potential* is equal to, or superior to, that of the male. If we consider that the female may have a more efficient heat-regulating system than the male, and that the highly trained female endurance runner can achieve cardio-vascular endurance capacities similar to those of the top male long-distance runners, it is not inconceivable that a woman could equal or even beat a man in marathon events.

As already mentioned, the female take-over in long-distance sea swimming has already occurred, although the physiological (biological) reasons for female supremacy in this event are different. Heat preservation is all important in cold water sea swimming. So, perhaps, the female heat regulating system is more efficient in *retaining* heat as well as *losing* it.

Rigorous Examination Shows 'Orthodox View' Held Because of Sociological and Psychological Factors

Assuming the validity of the argument I have put forward, the hypothesis I now propose is that, far from there being inherent biological and physiological reasons why the 'orthodox view' ought to be held as true, the reasons it is (incorrectly) held sociological. I have shown that the *belief* that there are fixed and immutable, innate biological factors that necessarily limit female sporting potential, and are the underlying reason for her inferiority in sporting performance, is false.

A distinction needs to be drawn between beliefs and attitudes. To clarify, consider, for instance, a proposal to devalue the pound sterling: let us suppose that we have two economists whose *beliefs* concerning this proposal are exactly the same. They are in full agreement as to what it is that is proposed, and also as to what in fact would be the economic, social and political consequences of adopting the proposal or, alternatively, of rejecting it. It is still possible – one may think it unlikely, but it seems to be possible – that notwithstanding this full agreement, their *attitudes* towards the proposal should differ; while agreeing exactly as to what the proposal is and would imply, one might be in favour of it, the other against. The distinction is perfectly clear. Beliefs are propositional and can be shown to be true or false, whilst attitudes are non-propositional and therefore can only be asserted to be right or wrong. In an ideal world a set of beliefs does ideally entail an attitude. So a *true* belief would entail a *right* attitude. In an ideal world, showing a set of beliefs to be false would be sufficient to transform the associated attitudes.

I hope I have shown that the 'orthodox view' is wrong because it is based on false beliefs. But, alas, our world is not perfect, and this alone is insufficient to transform the 'orthodox view'.

The attitudes which are an integral part of the 'orthodox view' are a function, not only of a false set of beliefs, but of layer upon layer of cultural bigotry that can be traced back in history to man's cultural origins. The reason the 'orthodox view' is held is not rational or logical. Rather, it is a specific example of the generally held attitude to women and the role they occupy in society. No amount of studies, the results of which would demonstrate that a set of beliefs were false, would suffice in transforming the attitudes. Analogously, a racist is a racist. When his beliefs about black inferiority are proved false, he is still a racist, because his racism is irrational and cannot be transformed by rational means.

No amount of studies illustrating that commonly held beliefs about women's abilities are false will change the all-pervading attitude of some people that women are inferior in sporting potential.

What is needed is a 'Gestalt switch'. I want to urge that people start by *assuming* real equality instead of waiting for studies to *prove* that there is equality. Equality in sporting potential, like other equalities, should be presupposed rather than something entailed by a set of beliefs. This insight justifies taking any steps to effect a switch in the basic attitudes to women. The attitude is irrational, so reason alone will never change it.

As the attitude cannot be changed by reason, it has to be eradicated, or fought, or resisted, or suppressed, until it withers away. A perfect example of this process is contained in the story of the women's marathon. A few women in the late 1960s in the United States tried to enter the Boston Marathon, purportedly an 'open' event. In 1967, one runner, Kathy Switzer, entered officially without revealing her sex. When it was discovered after the start that a woman was competing, race officials tried to eject her. They were unsuccessful and she became the first woman in history to compete *officially* in a marathon. The Amateur Athletic Union (AAU) of the United States immediately passed a ruling prohibiting competition between men and women, which meant that no women were allowed to run officially in marathons. It took 5 years of struggle and threats of court action, for the AAU to reverse its decision. The fruit of that battle is that today it is a commonplace to find women running the marathon.

If, as I have argued, there are no biological and physiological reasons for holding the view that women are necessarily inferior in sporting potential, the answers to women's inferiority hitherto in most sporting performances are to be found not so much in the natural sciences but more in the social sciences. *Dyer* [1976] investigated the social influences on female athletic and swimming performance. He identified the social factors as differential provision of facilities and encouragement of sport by education authorities, employers and the public at large in a number of countries; *Dyer* [1976] compared men and women's performances in these countries. As genetic and environmental factors in any one country would have equal relevance to males and females in that country, differences between the relative levels of achievement of men and women in different countries would seem to be an indication of the operation of more subtle social factors. For instance, women in different countries might be encouraged differentially, and have different expectation of their potential and abilities. These factors would influence their participation and hence their achievement levels.

In track events, *Dyer* [1976] calculated the percentage differences between male and female performances from national records in 1974 for 15 different countries. He found that the differences between the countries were large, with East Germany and the USSR heading the list, whilst France and Belgium were at the bottom. He concluded that these differences between countries were closely related to social and political structure, but were not very closely related to the level of male athletic performance. He suggests that the differences are due mainly to the differing expectations of women's achievements in different countries which in turn create differing levels of female participation, differing training regimes, and different social rewards for competing. Women's sport in the GDR is a social norm, whilst in France it is an aberration, for the most part.

In swimming, *Dyer* [1976] found that the female national records for one or more countries of the ten he investigated exceeded the male national records in one or more of the other countries. Indeed, he claims quite reasonably that Australian women swimmers would beat New Zealand men swimmers. He concludes that in swimming too, social factors are strongly influencing female performance.

If women in a country where participation in sport is encouraged and rewarded can produce performances of a calibre that surpass the top men in another country, it is not unreasonable to suggest that sociological factors are at work. If the social attitude to women in sport is to demean, discourage and undermine them, it is hardly surprising that the standards of female performance remain low. Facilities will be scarce, competition hard to find, and social derogation hard to bear.

In the GDR, women's participation in sport is of national importance, and consequently receives social approbation and approval along with superb opportunities for competition and training. The result is that the level of female performance is extremely high and approaches that of the men.

Furthermore, I propose that the 'orthodox view' itself has been, and still is, a primary contributing factor in preventing women from achieving their maximum sporting performances. A cultural milieu in which the belief is that women are incapable *by virtue of being women,* of performing certain activities, creates the conditions in which women are not able to perform those activities.

Unfortunately, in the field of sport, social prejudices exist that create psychological barriers which prevent women from even taking part in sport, let alone achieving their maximum performances. A study of school-leavers in Britain [*Emmett*, 1971] revealed that 60% of girls played no sport outside school, compared with 30% of boys; nearly half the girls interviewed planned to stop participating in sport completely on leaving school compared with less than a fifth of the boys.

At puberty, the cultural demands made on a young girl quite suddenly change at the time of the first menstruation. Parental control becomes more restrictive and society demands that the girl behaves in a way that conforms to a feminine sex-role stereotype. Her social acceptance as a woman, and hence her self-esteem, depend on her manifestations of her femininity [*Bardwick and Douvan*, 1971].

Although a young girl may be unclear about what to do in order to be a woman, she does respond to one single, clear directive, which is to withdraw from what is obviously designated masculine. Sport clearly falls into this category. Hence, unless an adolescent girl has the supportive family and social environment to counteract these cultural influences, she will probably choose to opt out of sport at school, using as often as she can her menstrual periods as a bona fide excuse. Perhaps, most importantly for my argument, avoiding sport and games is considered normal in teenage girls, and the collaboration that they receive from their parents and teachers is a testimony to the widespread social attitudes that prevail concerning women's sporting participation. This is the cultural context in which, for the most part in Western countries, women take part in sport.

History surrounding not just sport, but anything to do with female achievement, reveals that women themselves have a psychological barrier which prevents them from believing that they can achieve and succeed. As *Bardwick and Douvan* [1971] say: 'The essence of the problem of role conflict lies in the fact that... very few women have succeeded in traditionally masculine roles, not only because of disparagement and prejudice, but largely because women have not been fundamentally equipped and determined to succeed.' But the origins of this psychological barrier to success as *Bardwick and Douvan* [1971] intimates, lie in the traditional social role ascribed to women in which success-orientation has no part, *not* in some inherent feminine psychological trait that renders women innately incapable of achieving or succeeding.

Even our top sportswomen, who have weathered the negative sociocultural attitudes to their participation, and have reached the pinnacle of success in their event, are subject to the 'orthodox view'. Greta Waitz (Norway), whose 1980 world record time for the women's marathon of 2:25:40 would have won her every Olympic men's marathon up to 1948, has said: 'I don't think a woman can run a marathon as fast as a man. Physically men are stronger than we are.' This is a widely held belief amongst women runners. Not only are they holding false *beliefs* about themselves and their capacities, but more importantly, they are holding wrong *attitudes* about themselves and their capabilities.

The mental aspect of sport is universally accepted as crucially important, and can never be undersestimated. If women athletes themselves have the attitude that they are necessarily incapable of achieving a certain performance level, then this will act as a psychological barrier to their success in producing that performance.

So we see that the 'orthodox view', which I have attempted to undermine in this paper, is held not only by the general public, but by the top women athletes themselves, and has been and still is a primary contributing factor in preventing women from achieving their maximum sporting performances.

Summary

The orthodox view about women in sport is that, when compared with males, females have always and will always hold an inferior position in sporting achievement. The reason given is that there are biological factors that necessarily limit female performance potential. An examination of data from female sporting performance and of studies of physiological function in response to exercise provides evidence that refutes the 'orthodox view'. It is suggested, therefore, that the reasons the 'orthodox view' is held to be true are sociological and psychological rather than biological. Furthermore, it is argued that these psychosocial factors act as barriers to women achieving their maximum sporting performances.

References

Bardwick, J.M.; Douvan, E.: Ambivalence: the socialization of women; in Gornick, Moran, Woman in sexist society, pp. 225–241 (Mentor, New York 1971).

Brown, C.H.; Wilmore, J.H.: The effects of maximal resistance training on the strength and body composition of women athletes. Med. Sci. Sports 6: 133–138 (1974).

Burke, E.J.; Brush, F.C.: Physiological and anthropometric assessment of successful teenage female distance runners. Res. Quart. 50: 180–187 (1979).

Costill, D.L.; Bowers, R.; Kammer, W.F.: Skinfold estimates of body fat among marathon runners. Med. Sci. Sports 2: 93–95 (1970).

Costill, D.L.; Branham, G.; Eddy, D.; Sparks, K.: Determinants of marathon running success. Int. Z. angew. Physiol. 29: 249–254 (1971).

Cunningham, D.A.; Hill, J.S.: Effect of training on cardiovascular response to exercise in women. J. appl. Physiol. 39: 891–895 (1975).

Drinkwater, B.L.: Physiological responses of women to exercise; in Wilmore, Exercise and sport sciences reviews, vol. I, pp. 125–153 (1973).

Dyer, K.F.: Social influences on female athletic performance. J. biosoc. Sci. 8: 123–136 (1976).

Dyer, K.F.: The trend of the male-female performance differential in athletics, swimming and cycling 1948–1976. J. biosoc. Sci. 9: 325–338 (1977).

Edwards, M.A.: The effects of training at predetermined heart rate levels for sedentary college women. Med. Sci. Sports 6: 14–19 (1974).

Emmett, I.: Youth and leisure in an urban sprawl, pp. 29–38 (Manchester University Press, Manchester 1971).

Ferris, E.: Exploding the male myth. Sunday Telegraph (6th November 1977).

Ferris, E.: Sportswomen and medicine: the myths surrounding women's participation in sport and exercise. I and II. Olympic Rev. 138/139: 249–254; 140: 332–339 (1979).

Flint, M.M.; Drinkwater, B.L.; Horvath, S.M.: Effects of training of women's response to submaximal exercise. Med. Sci. Sports 6: 89–94 (1974).

Hertig, B.A.; Belding, H.S.; Kraning, K.K.; Batterton, D.L.; Smith, C.E.; Sargent, F., II: Artificial acclimatization of women to heat. J. appl. Physiol. 18: 383–386 (1963).

Kilbom, A.: Physical training in women. Scand. J. clin. Lab. Invest. 28: suppl. 119, pp. 1–34 (1971).

Lietzke, M.H.: An analytical study of world and Olympic racing records. Science 119: 333 (1954).

Lloyd, B.B.: The energetics of running; an analysis of world records. Adv. Sci. 22: 515 (1966).

Morimoto, T.; Slabochova, Z.; Norman, R.K.; Sargent, F.: Sex differences in physiological reactions to thermal stress. J. appl. Physiol. 22: 526–532 (1967).

Roskamm, H.: Optimum patterns of exercise for healthy athletes. Can. med. Ass. J. 96: 895–899 (1967).

Weinman, K.P.; Slabochova, Z.; Bernauer, E.M.; Morimoto, T.; Sargent, F., II: Reactions of men and women to repeated exposure to humid heat. J. appl. Physiol. 22: 533–538 (1967).

Wells, C.L.: Sexual differences in heat stress response. Physician Sportsmed. 5: 79–90 (1977).

Wilmore, J.H.: Alterations in strength, body composition and anthropometric measurements consequent to a 10-week weight training program. Med. Sci. Sports 6: 133–138 (1974).

Wilmore, J.H.: The application of science to sport: physiological profiles of male and female athletes. Can. J. appl. Physiol. 27: 25–31 (1979).

Wilmore, J.H.; Brown, C.H.: Physiological profiles of women distance runners. 6: 178–181 (1974).

Wilmore, J.H.; Brown, C.H.; Davis, J.A.: Body physique and composition of the female distance runner. Ann. N.Y. Acad. Sci. 301: 764–776 (1977).

Wyndham, C.H.; Morrison, J.F.; Williams, C.G.: Heat reactions of male and female Caucasians. J. appl. Physiol. 20: 357–364 (1965).

Dr. E.A.E. Ferris, 32 Addisland Court, Holland Villas Road, London W14 8DA (England)

Medicine Sport, vol. 15, pp. 30–40 (Karger, Basel 1981)

Women and Sport: A Leisure Studies Perspective[1]

M.J. Talbot

Trinity and All Saints' College, Horsforth, Leeds, England;
Centre for Urban and Regional Studies, University of Birmingham, England

Academic Approaches

Published academic study on female sports participation has tended to focus upon perceived value conflicts and anomalies in sex role; and on opportunities, constraints and supportive or inhibitory factors, both in the socialization process and in sports institutions. Less attention has been given to the relationship *between* women (participant and non-participant) and sport. It can be argued that knowledge of and insight into the problems shared by all women or by large numbers of women provide understanding, in social terms, of many of the problems encountered, not only by international sportswomen, but by sportswomen at many levels of commitment and achievement.

Thus, the study of the relationship between women and sport gains much from being placed in the wider context of general patterns of social and leisure behaviour, rather than being viewed solely from the rather narrow confine of sports sociology. Attention in this way is removed from the value conflicts between sports participation and femininity (so often seen as inevitable) and towards the experience (or non-experience) of sport by women within their social and demographic milieux, using the approaches and insights of the social sciences in a leisure studies perspective.

[1] The author wishes to thank the Dorette Wilkie Fund (Chelsea College of Physical Education Old Students' Association) for financial assistance to attend the congress.

An excellent critique of sports sociology as 'androcentric' is provided by *Hall* [1978], who suggests that sport itself possesses a gender – a masculine one – and that sports sociologists have largely ignored the feminist perspective, which she sees as 'dedicated to bringing women into the sociological imagination'. She makes the point, however, that there is danger, in concentrating on research in the area of women's experience, of 'intellectual ghettoization', and that the *male* gender role must not be ignored.

This danger would seem to be exacerbated by the fact that sports sociology itself could be described as sometimes insular and separatist in its approach, so leading, in the case of the study of women and sport, to artificially created schisms between women and men, and between sport and the rest of society, and preventing knowledge being integrated and socially meaningful. The criticism of the isolated study of women *in* sport and of women *and* sport, without consideration of the panorama of women's lives, is a valid one.

A further limitation of sports sociology as a framework for the study of women and sport is that it has tended to exclude or ignore consideration of the time constraint and various other structural factors, which have been identified by time budget researchers [*Szalai*, 1973, 1975] and by *Emmett* [1971] as crucial components of her 'social filter in the leisure field'. *Berlioux* [1978] has underlined the importance of women having limited free time in terms of the relative absence of women in the power structures of sport; and its influence on other processes of decision making should not be ignored.

The tendency, too, for sports sociology to focus only upon sportswomen who have achieved a high standard of performance or achievement, rather than on women who have rejected or been prevented participation, tends to produce an 'isolationist' or 'elitist' approach which implicitly ignores the problems of many women.

This paper is not intended to be a critique of sports sociology, but to provide a basis for the recognition that sociology as a discipline is *not* enough to begin to understand the complex relationships between men, women and sport. *Haworth and Smith* [1975] point out that an active view of man and woman requires interdisciplinary dialogue. They write: 'The dangers of non-cooperation may be very considerable. Discipline and specialist centred knowledge can result in decisions being taken without adequate appraisal of the causes, nature and consequences of problems. Human and financial costs can be high, especially if decisions become embedded in policies and plans affecting large groups and areas of social life.'

Leisure Studies

Since sport may be placed in the context of leisure (even where sport is a profession, since professional sport presupposes the existence of a leisured spectator or gambling group), it would therefore seem appropriate to use some of the concepts and insights developed within the rapidly emerging field of Leisure Studies. The eclectic use of the disciplinary 'human science' bases of geography, sociology, psychology, economics and anthropology, with foci on policy through family and community studies, social administration, and environmental, social and economic planning, provide useful items of knowledge and awareness which throw light on the essential relationships between men, women and sport.

In Britain the tendency towards multi- and inter-disciplinary work on leisure amongst academics has been complemented by the new awareness amongst existing research agencies that leisure is rapidly becoming a paramount consideration in people's lives. Thus, researchers in family and community studies, who had traditionally worked in multi- or inter-disciplinary teams, began to realize the crucial importance of leisure in their studies, and were able to bring their expertise and experience to bear on a subject which, hitherto, had tended to be studied in disciplinary compartments. This development has given rise to a whole cluster of concepts and ideas which leisure students can use to focus upon the particular problems or relationships in which they are interested. This has been true in the case of women and sport.

Difficulties of Studying 'Women' as a Group

The most immediately apparent difficulty in the study of women and sport is the very size of the population: women account for more than half the population of Great Britain and cannot be regarded as a homogeneous group. The differences between men and women with regard to sport behaviour are not as striking as the differences between different groups of women. When other parameters, such as social class and stage of life cycle, are added, these differences amongst women become even more marked. *Willis* [1974] has identified the task: '... not to measure these differences precisely and explain them physically, but to ask *why* some differences, and not others, are taken as so important, become so exaggerated, are used to buttress social attitudes or prejudice.'

To begin to fulfill this task, the interaction between women and sport needs to be seen in the context of the society in which it takes place. For this reason, most of the evidence which will be used in this paper will be from British sources, rather than North American sources, since it is clear that there exist different sets of constraints and opportunities in different societies.

Women as Leisure Servicer

Fundamental to the structure of contemporary western society is the complementary relationship of men and women, which also pervades sports and sports participation. Family studies [*Rapoport and Rapoport*, 1975; *Dumazedier*, 1967; *Fogarty* et al., 1971; *Leonard*, 1980] have supported the findings that women's leisure tends to be home-based and domestic by nature, and that this is even more marked in the early establishment phase of the family. It is at this stage more than any other that women's use of time seems to be predominantly a function of the needs (or demands) of their families. The function of women as 'servicers' to their families' leisure is reinforced by television advertisements (where washing powder X enables the mother to get her small son's football kit whiter than any other mother can; and perfume Y shows that she is a special kind of mother while she cheers on her son at school sports day) and is illustrated by the growing trend towards self-catering holidays, which assume the willingness of the mother to service the family.

Recognition of this servicing role to the family further underlines the complementary relationships between men, women, children and sport. It must be acknowledged that changes in women's own sport and leisure behaviour *necessarily* imply crucial changes in these complementary relationships. The part played by women in providing the support for men's and children's leisure activities requires further consideration, although reduction of such support in order to increase women's active participation could lead to domestic conflict and, as *Sharpe* [1976] concedes: '... many women draw much of their self esteem from their indispensability to their family. To deny this seems to remove the whole purpose of their existence.'

This dependence of family members on the maternal figure is illustrated by two recent accounts of mothers' commitment to their children's activities. *Toynbee* [1980], writing in the reflected glow of the Winter Olympics publicity this year, describes the way women transport their children to skating rinks for early morning and late night sessions: 'Lesser women might quail at the astonishing dedication of these skating mothers. They invest so much of their free time in their children that the rest of us could feel ashamed at not giving our children the same kind of undivided attention.'

Barker [1980], herself a physical education teacher, pictures the more often taken-for-granted servicing of activities by mothers: 'It is 11.30 p.m. and tears of tiredness run down my face as I hold out a rugby shirt to the fire in a desperate attempt to dry it before morning. ... I sometimes wonder whether *they* (physical education teachers) realize the effort that is put in by parents. I wouldn't mind an extra slip in the report books with a "well done" for me.'

This idea of women's leisure being, in effect, vicarious experience of their family's activity, legitimated by the service they provide, may go some way towards explaining the differential leisure behaviours of men and women, particularly in a traditional conjugal role relationship.

Family Studies

The theorists who observe a gradual change from 'traditional' to 'democratic' marriage role relationships would argue that the 'democratic' marriage 'releases the wife for leisure' [*Bell and Healey*, 1973], but this tempting thesis is not borne out by time budget research or by social surveys and family studies. Even the study entitled 'The Symmetrical Family' [*Young and Wilmott*, 1973] recognized the privatized nature of women's leisure.

The concept of social networks, developed within family studies and used extensively in community and leisure studies, can be adapted as 'supportive networks', in order to throw light upon the dependence of female sports participants on a supportive network, provided usually by husbands or female kin. The reasons for the presence of such support may be a function of the participant's commitment, or of shared interests, or of 'contractual understandings' with a marriage partner, or of the family's focussing of social contacts on the wife's participation. This phenomenon further underlines the need to understand more fully the complementary nature of conjugal roles or role constellations and the degree of reciprocality experienced, particularly by marriage partners. Indeed, the family research findings would suggest that, as the 'social chairmen' and culture bearers of their families, responsible as they are for the maintenance of contacts between different branches of their own and their husbands' families, married women tend to follow *family* leisure patterns, with only men and a few, more privileged women enjoying the supportive networks and freedom to follow individuated leisure patterns.

Life Cycle Approach

The recognition that domestic age or life cycle stage interacts dynamically with gender to influence leisure participation, has led to the use of the life cycle approach, where characteristic preoccupations are seen as sources of the salience of interests and activities. *Rapoport and Rapoport* [1975] in particular have used this approach to develop ideas about changing relationships between people and activities. They remark on the 'foreshortened perspective' of young girls, who see no further than marriage, and they note that differences between men and women, in the meaning of work outside the home, are more marked after the birth of children. The idea of 'career' is less common amongst women than men, and this difference can be observed, not only with regard to work, but also with regard to leisure activities. These findings have obvious relevance for the consideration of the salience of leisure activities for women at different stages of the life cycle.

It is all too easy for researchers and students to become 'blinkered' by their interest in a particular problem or phenomenon. There is a tendency thus to assume that it is *desirable and relevant* for women to take part in sport. The life cycle approach, by allowing, through retrospective or longitudinal study, consideration of the whole gamut of women's preoccupations, can disabuse the academic of this assumption. The work of *Leonard* [1980], for example, focusses on the period of courtship and marriage of couples in South Wales, this being the stage when so many girls and women in Britain drop out of active participation during leisure time. The tendency for the female peer group to collapse and for the girl to adopt her boyfriend's interests and friends until 'she has virtually no interests which are not courtship orientated' is in sharp contrast to the boy's continuing contact with and commitment to his peer group and activities, and places the relatively small amount of sports participation by girls firmly in a social context whose constraints are by no means exclusively related to the relationship between femininity and sport, or to structural and social barriers to participation.

Social Filter

It is important, however, to recognize the significance of these social and structural barriers – the two layers of mesh in the 'social filter' [*Emmett*, 1971]. The social barriers (and very real dangers) to young women going out alone, also mentioned by *Stanley* [1977], further emphasize the girl's dependence on her boyfriend or fiance. Our own research [*Talbot*, 1980] indicates that some girls actually enlarge their social and leisure contacts when they establish a firm relationship with a boy, and especially increase their ability to travel further afield. The natural reluctance of parents to allow girls the same freedom and mobility enjoyed by their brothers (ex-ampled by the motor bike!) begins in early childhood, and contributes towards the tendency to a future home-based life – excluding sport. The fact that a woman rarely has access to the family car [*Hillman and Whalley*, 1977], *if* she can drive, and the findings of the studies on isolated, house-bound women [*Gavron*, 1966; *Hobson*, 1978; *Parry and Johnson*, 1974; *Pearson*, 1976] emphasize the structural barriers to participation encountered by large numbers of the female population, through the family, finance, power and the law.

Time

There is no doubt, however, that the single greatest barrier to female participation in leisure activities is lack of time. 'The inordinately small amounts of free time at the disposal of employed women and the constraints put on the housewives' life are two factors which bear a heavy responsibility for women's reduced participation in civic life, in professional training, and education, etc. The implications for women's social advancement and pro-fessional career are quite obvious' [*Szalai*, 1975].

It would seem that, even when women are free *from* domestic and other commitments, they may not be free *to* do what they choose, because of they way in which their free time is perceived as *accountable* by their families. Further, the location and occurrence of their free time are often not suffi-ciently predictable to allow the time to be planned for. It is clear, from time budget research, that married couples do not share household tasks equally: there is convincing evidence that it is the wives who suffer from overload. *Hobson* [1978] describes the way in which some husbands allow their wives no *right* to leisure – their home and domesticity *are* their existence and their reward.

Class

The cut-off in leisure activity by working class girls has been reported by several researchers, and is also a function of working class girls' *real need* to find a marriage partner through their leisure activities, which then cease at marriage or before, because of their association with the search for a husband. The fact that physical prowess is deliberately excluded from the ethos of girls in youth cultures, as a juxtaposition to its place in boys' youth culture, highlights the need for more research on the place of girls in youth culture, in spite of the difficulties described by *McRobbie* [1978]: '... there is something about their culture which shuns outside interference of any sort, and this, I would argue, is gender specific. Unlike the boys at the youth club who played football and table tennis with the male youth leaders, the girls guarded their free time and privacy jealously and consistently refused to join in "official" club activities.'

Meanings

One area which has been relatively neglected by leisure research, but not by sports sociology, has been the agencies of socialization 'into' activities, which again display striking differences between boys and girls. Using a central concept from leisure studies, I have argued [*Talbot*, 1979] that sports may have different sets of *meanings* for males and females and that it may be difficult for girls, in the absence of supporting socializing agents, ever to 'know' physical activities well enough to achieve intrinsic satisfaction from them. The differential sets of interests between men and women found by the recent Leisure Provision and Human Need study [Institute for Family and Environmental Studies, 1978] and the frequently expressed wish (69% 'often' or 'frequently') that respondents' spouses shared more interests with them (sport accounting for 17% of non-shared interests) would support the idea that sport can be as *dysfunctional* in the family as it is satisfying for the individual, and that in many cases sport provides a human tragedy of non-communication between the sexes. I would argue that this non-communication is the greatest social *problem* associated with women and sport.

Problem Approach

Much of the writing on women and sport has been undertaken in response to the definition of sportswomen as a *problem,* in terms of the perceived conflict between femininity and sports achievement. The 'problem' area is even more confusing when one observes that, in leisure studies in general, and in policy making, it has been the female *non*-participant who has been defined as the problem!

It is necessary to know far more about *why* subjects are defined as problems, and *by whom* (in terms of the value positions of the definers), and whether those subjects see themselves or their behaviour as problematic. *Douglas* [1966] writes: 'It is not the act itself which has absolute value, but the social classification of it.' She suggests five solutions which society has found to the problem of anomaly; it is not difficult to find examples of each in relation to women and sport:

Douglas	Examples
1 Place it in a category and deny its other attributes	'Housewives aren't interested in sport'
2 Remove the anomaly by physical control	Women are not allowed in many sports pavilions, club houses and golf courses at peak times
3 Avoid the anomaly as abhorrent	'Contact sports are not ladylike' or even 'International sportswomen must be lesbians'
4 See the anomaly as highly dangerous and not to be associated with	The claim that strenuous activity harms women's reproductive functions: 'it's not natural' (for girls to play football) – actual statement by Ted Croker, Secretary of the Football Association [*Howe*, 1978]
5 Use ambiguous symbols in poetry, mythology and ritual	The recurrent theme of 'Amazons' in literature and poetry; the 'St. Trinian's' image of hockey players; the Tamara Press stereotype of field event female athletes

Such an analysis allows us to recognize attempted rationalisations for what they are, instead of allowing them to masquerade as *rationale* or *rational*.

Douglas [1966] also points out that society defines many phenomena as anomalous or problematic, and that these phenomena can be understood only in their social contexts, never in isolation. The predictions that society is developing towards a technologically based age of leisure make it even more desirable to recognize that female sports participation should be seen within the wider patterns of women's social and leisure behaviour. It is to be hoped that the artificial and wasteful separation between sports sociology and leisure studies, observed at the International Conference on Women and Sport in London in 1978, will not persist, so that useful and enlightening dialogue can be established between these two fields of study so relevant to women and sport.

'One half of the world cannot understand the pleasures of the other.'

Emma, Jane Austen

Summary

Fundamental to the structure of contemporary society is the complementary relationship between men and women, which also pervades sports and sports participation. Crucial changes in that complementary relationship are necessarily implied by changes in women's sport and leisure behaviour. It is argued that women's sports participation and involvement can be seen as a function of their wider patterns of leisure behaviour, rather than as an inevitable value conflict between femininity and sport. The social definitions of sportswomen *and* non-participants as 'problematic' are discussed in relation to societal values and systems.

References

Barker, P.: Pity the poor parent. Br. J. phys. Ed. *11:* 16 (1980).

Bell, C.; Healey, P.: The family and leisure; in Smith et al., Leisure and society in Britain (Lane, London 1973).

Berlioux, M.: Women in the Olympic context; in Central Council for Physical Recreation, Women in Sport. Proc. Int. Conf., London 1978.

Douglas, M.: Purity and danger (Routledge & Kegan Paul, London 1966).

Dumazedier, J.: Toward a society of leisure (New York, Free Press 1967).

Emmett, I.: The social filter in the leisure field. Recreation News, suppl. No. 4, Countryside Commission (1971).

Fogarty, M.P.; Rapoport, R.; Rapoport R.: Sex, career and family (Allen & Unwin, London 1971).

Gavron, H.: The captive wife (Penguin, London 1966).

Hall, M.A.: Sport and gender: a feminist perspective on the sociology of sport (Canadian Association for Health, Physical Education & Recreation, Ottawa 1978).

Haworth, J.; Smith, M.A. (eds): Work and leisure, p. 5 (Lepus, London 1975).

Hillman, M.; Whalley, A.: Fair play for all: a study of access to sport and informal recreation (Political and Economic Planning, London 1977).

Hobson, D.: Housewives: isolation as oppression. Women's studies group, Women Take Issue; Centre for Contemporary Cultural Studies (University of Birmingham/Hutchinson, London 1978).

Howe, Lady: A little too strenuous for women? In central council for physical recreation, women in sport, int. conf. London (1978).

Institute for Family & Environmental Studies/Dartington Amenity Research Trust: Leisure provision and human need: report on household survey, working paper No. 3 (London 1978).

Leonard, D.: Sex and generation: a study of courtship and weddings (Tavistock, London 1980).

McRobbie, A.: Working class girls and culture of femininity, in Women's Studies Group, Women Take Issue, p. 101 (Centre for Contemporary Cultural Studies, University of Birmingham, Birmingham/Hutchinson, London 1978).

Parry, N.C.A.; Johnson, D.: Leisure and social structure. Final report to Social Science Research Council, London (1974).

Pearson, L.: Working class non-work time: a case study in Birmingham; PhD thesis, Birmingham (1976).

Rapoport, R.; Rapoport, R.: Leisure and the family life cycle (Routledge & Kegan Paul, London 1975).

Sharpe, S.: Just like a girl: how girls learn to be women, p. 54 (Penguin, London 1976).

Stanley, L.: Sex, gender and the sociology of leisure; in Smith, Leisure and urban society (Leisure Studies Association, Manchester 1977).

Szalai, A.: The use of time: daily activities of urban and suburban populations in twelve countries (Mouton, The Hague 1973).

Szalai, A.: Women's time: women in the light of contemporary time budget research. Futures 7: 385–399 (1975).

Talbot, M.J.: Meaning in physical activity: a speculative discussion. Momentum 4: 28–33 (1979).

Talbot, M.J.: Women's leisure behaviour, with particular reference to physical activity; current PhD thesis, Birmingham (1980).

Toynbee, P.: Guardian Women. The Guardian, London (Jan. 28, 1980).

Willis, P.: Performance and meaning – a socio-cultural view of women in sport. Cult. Stud. 5: 21–36 (1974).

Young, M.; Wilmott, P.: The symmetrical family (Routledge & Kegan Paul, London 1973).

M.J. Talbot, MA, 53 Windmill Lane, Yeadon, Leeds LS19 7TQ (England)

Medicine Sport, vol. 15, pp. 41–48 (Karger, Basel 1981)

The Influence of the Traditional Sex Roles on Women's Participation and Engagement in Sport

K. Fasting, J.O. Tangen

The Norwegian College of Physical Education and Sport, Oslo, Norway

Introduction

Under Norwegian law women and men have the same legal rights. However, a norwegian study, concerning living conditions has shown that women compared to men are rated lower in several areas, and have fewer opportunities than men [*NOU*, 1976, p. 28]. These were basic living conditions such as education, free time at one's disposal, admission to gainfully employed work, freedom to choose occupation, opportunity to take active part in community life, and the possibility to influence one's own life. Antecedent constraining factors have also influenced peoples' participation and engagement in sports activities [*Fasting*, 1980]. Consequently, women's possibilities to be engaged in sport are fewer than men's.

The meaning of equality must be that both sexes have the same social, mental, and physical possibilities to participate in all areas of community life according to one's own wishes, needs and expectations. Since sport is one of the most attractive leisure-time activities of today, it is important that true equality also exists in this area.

Purpose

Society is still ruled by men. This male domination is more clear in the world of sports than in other areas in the society. Norms and values of the 'traditional' male role define both the organization of, and behavior in, sports. According to traditional roles, desirable qualities for males in our culture are aggressiveness, independency, and achievement. Females on the

Table I. Physical activity among gainfully employed men and women, and housewives

Activity level	Gainfully employed men		Gainfully employed women		Housewives	
	n	%	n	%	n	%
Passive	339	33	141	33	364	46
Active	679	67	282	67	435	54
Total	1,018	100	423	100	799	100

$X^2 = 32.83$; d.f. $= 2$; p $= < 0.001$; $\Phi = 0.12$.

other hand should be submissive, dependent, emotional, illogical, affectionate, and not too intelligent [*Ward and Balswick*, 1978; *Sage and Loudermilk*, 1979; *Hall*, 1972].

Traditionally, sports and vigorous physical activities have been positively associated with the male role and negatively associated with the female role [*Harris*, 1975; *Felshin*, 1974; *Hart*, 1976; *Soutar*, 1979]. *Butt* [1976, p. 68] put it this way: 'When judged within a traditional framework of social values, the woman pursuing an athletic career is pursuing a male role. The role of athlete and the role of female are opposed.' The 'traditional' male role and the sport role have consequently much more in common than the sport role and the 'traditional' female role. Therefore, it is more natural for men than women to engage in sports. *Holter* [1970] has shown that women's attitudes towards sex role norms varies with their occupational status. Housewives not gainfully employed display a much more traditional attitude to the sex role norms than housewives gainfully employed full-time. We may therefore expect that gainfully employed women are much closer to the male and sport role than housewives. They may therefore be more involved in sports than housewives, but still less than men.

The purpose of this paper is to test the following two hypotheses: (1) Gainfully employed men are more involved in sports than gainfully employed women. (2) Gainfully employed women are more involved in sports than housewives.

Three dimensions of involvement were measured. These were physically active versus passive, member versus non-member of a sports club, and participation versus non-participation in competitive sports. People were considered more involved if they, in addition to being physically active,

Table II. Membership in sports clubs among gainfully employed men and women, and housewives

Membership	Gainfully employed men		Gainfully employed women		Housewives	
	n	%	n	%	n	%
Yes	301	30	62	15	74	9
No	705	70	356	85	712	91
Total	1,006	100	418	100	786	100

$X^2 = 124.89$; d.f. $= 2$; p $= < 0.001$; $\Phi = 0.24$.

were also a member of a sports club. The most involved in sport were those who were physically active, a member of a sports club, and participated in competitive sports [*Kinrell*, 1976].

Procedure

The data material used were part of a nationwide study on participation and interest in physical activity among the Norwegian population. The study took place in 1973 and 3,100 persons above 15 years of age were personally interviewed. People living on a pension, pupils, students, and military conscripts are excluded in this particular study, and the results are therefore based on a sample of 2,240 persons.

Results

In leisure time, 67% of gainfully employed women and men participated in different forms of physical activity. Housewives were less physically active (table I). Concerning time spent in physical activity per month, the means for the three occupational groups were respectively 347, 323, and 306 min. While 30% of gainfully employed men were members of a sports club, only 15% among gainfully employed women and 9% among the housewives had a similar membership (table II). One fourth of the sample had been more physically active 5 years ago. The reasons for their reduction in sport participation are shown in table III.

Two answers were of special interest to our hypotheses. They were: 'no family responsibility then' and 'more time available in the past'. While

Table III. Reasons for being more active 5 years ago among gainfully employed men and women, and housewives

Reasons	Gainfully employed men		Gainfully employed women		Housewives	
	n	%	n	%	n	%
No family responsibility	24	10	21	17	40	21
Younger	66	28	27	21	78	41
More time available	65	28	30	24	33	17
More interested	23	10	16	13	8	4
Better environmental stimulation	11	5	4	3	7	4
Better opportunities	22	10	14	11	9	5
In school	11	5	9	7	7	4
Something else	10	4	5	4	8	4
Total	232	100	126	100	190	100

$X^2 = 37.49$; d.f. $= 14$; p $= < 0.001$; $\Phi^1 = 0.19$.

only 10% of employed men claimed that family responsibility was a reason for being less active, 17% of gainfully employed women and 21% of housewives gave this as a reason.

About 17% of the gainfully employed men, versus 24% of gainfully employed women and 28% of the housewives said that they previously had more available time. Of the 2,240 persons 9% participated in sports competitions. The percentages of participation were respectively 16, 2, and 2 among gainfully employed men, women, and housewives. 650 persons had stopped participation in sports competition. Marriage was the most common reason among women. 43% of the housewives and 29% of employed women gave this answer. Only 8%, however, of the men claimed that marriage was the main reason for leaving sports competition. Marriage that included pregnancy and giving birth can be the reason for females to drop out from sport. The difference between the two female groups indicates that marriage not necessarily implies a permanent halt. Our opinion is that both parents should have equal responsibility in bringing up children. The influence of the traditional sex role pattern on participation in sports is clearly illustrated by the fact that only 8% of the men give marriage as a reason for leaving competitive sport.

Discussion

The results confirmed most of our expectations and hypotheses. We found, however, no differences in participation in physical activity in leisure time between gainfully employed men and women. However, this could be explained, as a result, by our very broad definition of the concept 'physical activity'. It includes all kinds of physical leisure-time activities, from traditional sports to hiking. It does not include working in the garden, car washing, etc., and physical activity in connection with transport to and from work. Studies have shown that the difference between the sexes concerning participation in sport is greater with a more restricted concept, for example if amount of time and frequency are controlled [*Fasting*, 1980].

The same tendency is shown in our study. The differences between the sexes are greater when the amount of time training is controlled and among people taking part in competitive sports. No difference in participation in sport competition was however found between the two groups of women. For housewives to be active in competitive sport probably implies a change of role and values far beyond that of their norms. The number of women participating in competitive sport, however, is very small, so no valid conclusions can be drawn.

The amount of leisure time may be one factor that influences people's participation in sports [*Robinson*, 1967; *Röblitz*, 1964]. Studies have shown, however, that gainfully employed women have less time to their own disposal than housewives [Central Bureau of Statistics, 1975; NOU 1976, p. 28]. In spite of this, gainfully employed women were found in our study to be more involved in sport than housewives.

Traditionally, the lower rate of the women's involvement in sport has been explained as a result of a cognitive dissonance and a role conflict they feel or anticipate between the 'traditional' female role and the sport role. In the tradition of cognitive consistency theories [*Abelson* et al., 1968], we may expect that women, in relation to sport participation, behave in a way that maximizes the internal consistency of their cognitive system.

As mentioned earlier the norms and values of the 'traditional female' role are in contrast to the sport role. Among women this phenomenon can result in an inter-role conflict. However, the severity of the conflict will vary with the types of sports since some subdisciplines are more accepted as 'feminine' than others. Only seldom will men experience such a conflict. Normally, participation in sport confirms the 'traditional masculine' role.

If such explanations as suggested here should be empirically verified, this would demand more extensive and in-depth studies than our survey. However, the results concerning withdrawal from sport participation in general and from competitive sport suggest that theories of cognitive consistency can be one explanation of this phenomenon. *Hall* [1978] questions this proposed role conflict and claims that: 'Although empirical research is negligible adult female athletes do not perceive role conflict, and in general appear to be quite pleased with their life-styles.' It should be noticed that most of the studies in this area concern women who already are involved in sports [*Snyder and Kivlin*, 1975; *Snyder* et al., 1975; *Snyder and Spreitzer*, 1976; *Harris and Jennings*, 1977]. *Sage and Loudermilk* [1979] found, however, that female athletes participating in sports which have been traditionally not socially approved, experienced significantly greater role conflict than those participating in more socially approved sports. Whether female *athletes* experience a role conflict or not is not the interesting question here. Instead we may ask whether this anticipated role conflict obstructs women entering sports. We may also ask if such a role conflict, conscious or unconscious, can explain women's drop out from sport?

This low involvement and drop out may also be seen from another point of view. Many women do not engage in sport because of lack of interest. The sports world and its values do not appeal to them. Values that dominate the sports world do not fit within the culture of women. They prefer other leisure-time activities that fit their own values better.

The suggestions mentioned here can probably explain why women as a group are less active in sports than men. They can also explain why gainfully employed women are more involved in sports than housewives. They have modified their own values and their female role. Whether housewives do not engage in sport because of lack of interest or because of an anticipated role conflict, they are in both situations tied up in the 'traditional' female role [*Holter*, 1970].

Participating in physical activities and sports is important for fulfilling one's potentialities in our technical and industrial society. However, two conditions must be changed before we will have equality between men and women in sport. First of all the 'traditional' sex roles must be changed so that women do not feel or anticipate the role conflict. But it is also important that those values that dominate the women's culture can influence and change sport from inside.

As *Butt* [1976, p. 75] says: 'Women must influence and reform the sports system rather than be bought off by it.' If women's participation in sports is to be increased, they must be allowed to and encouraged to participate in defining the norms and values of sports. They must therefore be encouraged and given the practical possibilities to function at all administrative levels in the sports organizations.

Summary

2,240 persons were personally interviewed in a nationwide study about their involvement in sport. The results show that gainfully employed men were more involved in sport than gainfully employed women. However, gainfully employed women were more involved in sport than housewives. It was concluded that this was a result of an anticipated role conflict and a different value-orientation in the traditional culture of women.

References

Abelson, R.P.; Aronson, E.; McGuire, W.J.; Newcomb, T.M.; Rosenberg, M.J.; Tannenbaum, P.H.: Theories of cognitive consistency (RandMcNally, Chicago 1968).
Butt, S.D.: Psychology of sport, pp. 68–76 (Van Nostrand & Reinhold, New York 1976).
Central Bureau of Statistics: Tidsnyttingsundersøkelsen 1971–72, hefte 1 (Oslo 1975).
Fasting, K.: Fysisk aktivitet i fritiden (Norges idrettshøgskole, Oslo 1980).
Felshin, J.: The triple option . . . For women in sport. Quest 21: 36–40 (1974).
Hall, A.M.: A 'female women' and an 'athletic women' as viewed by female participants and non-participants in sport. Br. J. phys. Ed. 3: 43–46 (1972).
Hall, A.M.: Sport and gender: a feminist perspective on the sociology of sport (Cahper, Ottawa 1978).
Harris, D.: Psychological consideration. J. phys. Ed. Recr. 46: 32–36 (1975).
Harris, D.; Jennings, S.E.: Self-perception of female distance runners; in Milvy, The marathon: physiological, medical, epidemiological and psychological studies (New York Academy of Sciences, New York 1977).
Hart, M.: On being female in sport; in Hart, Sport in the sociocultural process; 2nd ed., pp. 291–303 (Brown, Iowa 1976).
Holter, H.: Sex roles and social structure (Universitetsforlaget, Oslo 1970).
Kinrell, J.: Ungdomars involvering i idrett (Mölndal, Ped. inst. Lärarhögskolan i Mölnda 1976).
NOU 1976: 28 Levekårsundersøkelsen, sluttrapport (Oslo 1976).
Robinson, J.P.: Time expenditure on sports across ten countries. Int. Rev. Sport Soc. 2: 67–84 (1967).
Röblitz, G.: Die sportliche Betätigung im Freizeitverhalten von Jugendlichen zwischen 17 und 18 Jahren. Theorie Prax. Körperkult. 13: 498–510 (1964).
Sage, G.H.; Loudermilk, S.: The female athlete and role conflict. Res. Quart. 1: 88–96 (1979).
Snyder, E.E.; Kivlin, J.E.: Women athletes and aspects of psychological well-being and body image. Res. Quart. 2: 191–198 (1975).

Snyder, E.E.; Kivlin, J.E.; Spreitzer, E.: The female athlete: analysis of objective and subjective role conflict; in Landers, Psychology of sport and motor behavior (Pennsylvania State University Press, University Park 1975).

Snyder, E.E.; Spreitzer, E.: Correlates of sport participation among adolescent girls. Res. Quart. 4: 804–809 (1976).

Soutar, A.J.: Women in society and sport: towards a closer understanding of the dilemma

facing female athletes. Momentum 2: 16–24 (1979).

Ward, D.; Balswick, J.: Strong men and virtuous women. Pacific Soc. Rev. 1: 45–55 (1978).

K. Fasting, Ass. Prof., The Norwegian College of Physical Education and Sport, PO Box 40, Kringsjaa, Oslo 8 (Norway)

Medicine Sport, vol. 15, pp. 49–57 (Karger, Basel 1981)

Personality Research:
Implications for Women in Sport

D.V. Harris

Center for Women and Sport, The Pennsylvania State University,
University Park, Pa., USA

Universally sports competition has been the prerogative of the male. It has been assumed that sports experience provided a laboratory for socializing the male for appropriate masculine behavior. Traditionally the behavioral demands in competitive sport reinforce what is stereotypically masculine and what the male is supposed to emulate in most societies. At the same time, the psychological and physical demands of sport are not generally considered compatible with any society's stereotyped image of femininity. The behavioral demands in sport are the antithesis of what the female is supposed to be. In many societies it has been to her detriment, behaviorally, to pursue serious involvement in competitive sports.

Almost without exception personality instruments perpetuate a double standard of behavior, one for females and one for males. Generalizing the results of the personality-competitive sports relationship among females, one would observe that the female athlete tends to differ significantly from the norm on many variables. She scores higher than the norm on such behaviors as self-confidence, self-control, personal adjustment, achievement, dominance, endurance, order, intraception, affiliation, exhibition, aggression, change, and other variables that would be necessary for success in competitive sport. On the other hand, she scores significantly lower than the norm on traits such as femininity, nurturance, succorance, abasement, and other behaviors that are traditionally accorded the stereotyped female.

When male and female athletes are scored on the same scales and compared to the male norms, their behaviors are more alike than different. This would suggest that behaviors that are demanded for successful participation in sports competition are not linked with one's sex. They are behaviors that human beings, male or female, must have to find the behavioral demands of the sports environment compatible with their own personality characteristics. Due to the traditional double standard of behavior, much of the research examining sex differences in personality must be disregarded or reinterpreted from a different perspective. Inasmuch as the personality characteristics of the stereotyped male are compatible with the behaviors needed for sport competition, it is not surprising to observe that females who find sport competition satisfying and challenging are behaviorally more like males who enjoy sport than they are like their stereotyped female peers.

Much of the research on the female athlete has consisted of comparisons to non-athletes or to female norms. This procedure has resulted in the generalized conclusion that sport 'masculinizes' the behavior of females. With the universal women's movement, a demand for better instruments with less bias has been made. For this reason, the following discussion will be devoted to new considerations and new dimensions of examining behaviors which will have implications for sport psychology with particular emphasis on the female athlete.

The physical differences between men and women are obvious and universal; the psychological differences are not. In spite of these acknowledged facts, people continue to hold strong beliefs about psychological sex differences even when those beliefs are not supported by scientific fact and research. Individuals are born either male or female; they must learn to be masculine or feminine.

In short, the two sexes learn most of their behavior with equal facility in a wide variety of situations. *Maccoby and Jacklin* [1974] concluded from a survey of literature that many popular beliefs about the psychological characteristics of the two sexes have little or no basis. In spite of this lack of evidence many people continue to believe and to perpetuate differences that do not exist. This is especially true with the female athlete.

As investigators begin to examine the female and her role in society and to sort out what is the product of one's socialization from the product of one's biological sex, it becomes more and more evident that characteristics previously considered sex related are culturally determined. The behavior of males, as well as females, is minimally dependent on biological differences and much more dependent upon the restricted position that both are channeled into in today's society. Parents and society teach children to be boys and girls by rewarding them for appropriate sex-role behavior and punishing cross-gender behavior. *Marmor* [1973] said that gender role and gender identity, although generally related to the biological sex of a child, actually are not shared by biological factors but by cultural ones. Once a child's biological ascription is settled, a myriad of culturally defined cues begin to be presented to the developing infant which are designed to shape its gender identity to its assigned sex. While boys get reinforced by building a concept of self-esteem based on accomplishments which are tangible and objective, the girls learn not to gratify impulses that adults find offensive and to rely on others to determine whether they have done well or poorly in any given situation. Girls learn to please, to defer, to wait for reinforcement. This becomes a part of being 'feminine'.

The difference in attitudes and acceptance towards males and females in sport originates in the differences in traits that society ascribes to each sex. *Kagan and Moss* [1962], basing their definitions on observations and research during a longitudinal study of children, described the traditional masculine model as athletic, active sexually, independent, dominant, courageous, and competitive. The female was described as passive and dependent, socially anxious, sexually timid, and fearful of problem situations. *Douvan and Adelson* [1966] labeled the females who said that they felt more important and useful when they were participating in competitive sports and games as 'nonfeminine'. Only those girls who followed the traditional roles of expectations were considered 'normal'.

The etiology of negative sanctioning appears to be grounded in the notion that serious participation in athletics, by virtue of its physical and psychological demands, is incongruous with what is considered 'appropriate' feminine behavior. Somehow, it is as though the female has traded off her femininity to become an athlete. *Cheska* [1970] described a paradox when she indicated that the personality traits that are considered undesirable in the female include aggressiveness, independence, ambition, assertiveness, and having goals other than being a wife or mother. Yet, these are the specific traits needed by females if they are to succeed in attaining a different role or to play competitive sports. One can conclude, based on the available research, that the role conflict is a manifestation of dissonance between those behavioral characteristics necessary for success in athletics and those that are considered appropriate feminine behaviors. This conflict can produce a real identity crisis within the young female who is struggling to establish her own identity when she discovers that she enjoys participating in competitive sports and finds it challenging and satisfying. Traditionally, the female has resolved this conflict by withdrawing from sport during adolescence when her body begins to mature and she has her femaleness reinforced constantly.

Increasing numbers of females are now discovering that they can cope with any superimposed conflicts by adapting to the demands of the situation in which they find themselves. They are flexible enough behaviorally to function confidently in both sport and social situations without conflict. They do not feel that they have had to trade off their feminine self to be an athlete. Several investigators [*Beach*, 1974; *Kennicke*, 1972; *Monk*, 1976; *Snyder* et al., 1975] have reported that in spite of the notion that sports competition is not compatible with the expected sex-role orientation, the negative feedback the female athlete received as a result of violating this role did not adversely influence her self-perceptions. *Snyder* et al. [1975] reported that, on the contrary, positive relationships emerged in the opposite direction. They concluded that their findings raised serious doubts about the assumptions of the conflict being inherent in female athletes which might produce a negative self-perception.

The position that has dominated the writings and personality instruments of social and behavioral scientists is that masculine and feminine attributes are essentially bipolar opposites. The presence of feminine characteristics tends to preclude the appearance of masculine ones. Indeed, the absence of a feminine attribute is by definition, equivalent to masculinity. Conversely, masculine characteristics are assumed to preclude feminine ones and their absence is to define femininity.

Distinction between the sex-roles is universal among human societies; males are assigned different tasks, rights, and privileges, and are generally subject to different rules of conduct than females. Males and females are typically assumed to possess different temperamental characteristics and abilities whose existence is used to justify the perpetuation of a double standard of behavior. Definitive data are lacking about whether there are genetically determined differences in the temperamental make-up of males and females; however, there is abundant evidence to support the fact that the human personality is highly malleable.

Psychologists have tended to accept as given the complex set of sex-related phenomena and to focus attention on the processes of which individuals come to correspond in their behaviors and attributes to the expected norm for their sex within their culture. Psychologists have also been interested in the variability among individuals and have attempted to identify the factors that promote or interfere with the development of expected and appropriate patterns of behavior. Psychological inquiries have been based on the notion that the categorical variable of biological gender is intimately associated with masculine and feminine role behaviors and the presumed psychological differences between males and females. This bipolar conception of masculinity and femininity has historically been the one that has guided the research efforts of psychologists. It no longer appears to be an appropriate concept.

Helmreich and Spence [1977] contend that the relationship among the various components of masculinity and femininity such as biological gender, sex-roles, sexual orientation and especially psychological attributes of masculinity and femininity and the adoption of conventional sex-roles is not as strong as has been traditionally assumed. Their position represents the more contemporary concept that masculinity and femininity represent two separate dimensions which vary independently. *Helmreich and Spence* [1977] have developed a new instrument, the Personal Attributes Questionnaire (PAQ), to assess masculine-feminine components of behavior. While they have maintained the psychological aspects of masculinity and femininity, they have discarded a strictly bipolar model and structured an essentially dualistic concept.

The PAQ is composed of a masculinity and a femininity scale. The items on the masculinity scale include those attributes considered as socially desirable in both sexes but observed to a greater degree among males. Conversely, those attributes considered as socially desirable in both sexes but found to a greater extent among females constituted the femininity scale. Two scores are generated, one on each scale. An individual is classified according to his or her position relative to the scale medians. Individuals scoring above the median on both scales are classified as *androgynous*. Those scoring high on the masculine scale and below median on femininity scale are *masculine* while those scoring high on the femininity scale and below median on the masculinity scale are *feminine*. Those scoring below the median on both scales are considered *undifferentiated*.

Using several hundred subjects, *Helmreich and Spence* [1977] have studied the relationship between the two scales. They observed a tendency for high masculine scores to be associated with high feminine scores and low scores on one to be associated with low scores on the other. A bipolar conception would suggest that the sets of scores would be negatively related. If one has a high masculine score, the feminine score would be low; the authors did not find this negative relationship.

When examining the relationship of the behavioral frame of reference as assessed by the PAQ and self-esteem, *Spence* et al. [1975] reported that the lowest self-esteem was observed among the undifferentiated, next lowest among those classified as feminine, followed by masculine with the highest observed among the androgynous group. These data suggest that masculinity and androgyny are related to desirable behaviors and positive self-esteem in both males and females.

In an attempt to validate their findings *Helmreich and Spence* [1977] studied unique populations of females where the existence or nonexistence of differences in the distribution of masculinity and femininity might support their theoretical proposition. A group of female athletes was included and data from these women suggested that high achieving women are more likely to possess both masculine and feminine attributes than their male counterparts without suffering any deficit in their femininity. On the contrary, they displayed significantly higher self-esteem than those females who were classified as feminine in a traditional sense.

In a series of studies which began in 1976, *Harris and Jennings* [1977, 1978] have found no evidence to support the supposed, inevitable trade-off of the female athlete's self-esteem and femininity for making a serious commitment to sports participation. These studies indicated that it is not being male or female per se, or being an athlete, but the psychological attributes that provide the behavioral frame of reference which was related to self- esteem.

Further studies were conducted examining the relationship of motivation and one's behavioral frame of reference. Paradoxically, the one consistency in achievement motivation has been the inconsistency of results when females have been studied [*Karabenick and Marshall*, 1974; *Weiner* et al., 1971]. Among those researchers who chose not to ignore female subjects was *Mehrabian* [1969] who concluded that the inconsistent results were attributed to the possibility that different measures of achievement motivation are required for females and males. *Mehrabian* [1969], along with *Jackson* et al. [1976], have questioned a unitary concept of achievement motivation saying it is too simplistic and thus fails to have predictive validity in real-life settings.

Hypothesizing that some of the inconsistencies in the motivation literature could be attributed to its unitary conceptualization, *Spence and Helmreich* [1978] developed the Work and Family Orientation Scale (WOFO) to assess several components of achievement motivation. They were: (1) work – the desire to work hard and keep busy; (2) mastery – the desire to cope with challenging tasks and to meet inner standards of excellence; (3) competitiveness – reflecting a desire to win over other people; and (4) personal unconcern – being unconcerned with other's negative reactions to one's achievement. The WOFO was designed on the premise that the nature of achievement motivation is essentially the same in both sexes; therefore, a single set of scales could be applicable.

In a series of studies at Penn State, subjects completed both the PAQ and WOFO. In all analyses the classifications of androgynous, masculine, feminine, and undifferentiated were used as levels of one factor to examine the independent variables of mastery, work, competitiveness, and personal unconcern. In a population of females, androgynous individuals scored significantly higher than those classified as feminine and undifferentiated on the motivation components of mastery, work, and competitiveness. Masculine individuals scored significantly higher than feminine or undifferentiated individuals on the mastery scale. On the personal unconcern scale, female athletes differed significantly from their nonathletic peers in that they showed more concern about what others thought. However, upon closer examination of the results, female athletes classified as feminine were primarily responsible for the difference within the athletic population. This supported the hypothesis that traditional, stereotyped females would show greater concern about what others think because of their perceived conflict.

When male and female athletes were compared, those individuals classified as androgynous and/or masculine scored higher on mastery, work, and competitiveness with females scoring significantly higher than males on the work component. These results lend credence to the assumption that deficits in achievement motivation are at least partially explained by differences in the stereotypic characteristics associated with masculinity and femininity rather than gender.

In summary, increasing levels of understanding and changing attitudes about human behavior have indicated that the stereotyped masculine and feminine roles for males and females respectively are no longer appropriate for socializing human beings to function effectively in today's society. As a result, most of the personality instruments which perpetuate these stereotyped expectancies for male and female behavior are no longer appropriate. Their use should be discontinued, especially among female athletic populations. Males and females are very much alike psychologically. Many ways in which they differ can be explained by being socialized to meet stereotyped expectancies rather than by one's biology.

The behavioral demands of competitive sport are more dissonant with the stereotyped expectancies of feminine behavior. This explains why there has been more concern about the conflicts that female athletes may experience psychologically. With new ways of conceiving behavior, research is finding that male and female athletes are more similar than different in their behaviors.

Future research in the personality of athletes, both male and female, needs to demonstrate the preference for theory over unrelated collections of data. Preference for theories supported by data must also be shown; theory and data should complement each other. *Morgan* [1972] recommended to those who desire to study personality among female athletes to pursue it within a theoretical framework. From the outset appropriate instrumentation, sampling procedures, and statistical techniques should be utilized as an extensive normative data base is developed. Longitudinal studies accompanied with rigorous definitions on dependent and independent variables should be conducted. Hopefully, investigators will not commit the same methodological errors which have characterized the personality research of the male athlete. With increasing numbers of female athletes participating in sports throughout the world, there are sufficient opportunities to examine the personality of the female athlete (and the male athlete) in new, innovative, and creative ways that will incorporate new ways of conceiving behavior that are more appropriate in contemporary society. We certainly know very little about the personality of athletes at this point in time.

Summary

Personality research on female athletes is fraught with the same methodological problems and shortcomings as that involving male athletes. Prediction of athletic success has been the goal, however, that has never been realized. Existing results on female athletes are compounded by personality norms which reflect distinctions between masculine and feminine expectancies in behavior that are no longer appropriate. Traditionally masculine and feminine attributes have been viewed as bipolar opposites in psychological research. Since the 1970s several theorists maintain that masculinity and femininity are two separate dimensions: the manifestation of one neither logically nor psychologically precludes possession of the other. Implications for sport are discussed.

References

Beach, B.: Males' perceptions of highly skilled female participants; MS thesis, University Park (1974).

Cheska, A.: Current developments in competitive sports for girls and women. J.O.H.P.E.R. *41:* 86–91 (1970).

Douvan, E.; Adelson, J.: The adolescent experience (Wiley, New York 1966).

Harris, D.V.; Jennings, S.E.: Self-perception of female distance runners; in Milvy, The marathon: physiological, medical, epidemiological, and psychological studies (New York Academy of Sciences, New York 1977).

Harris, D.V.; Jennings, S.E.: Achievement motivation: there is no fear-of-success in female athletes. Paper presented Fall Conf. Eastern Ass. Physical Education of College Women, Hershey 1978.

Helmreich, R.; Spence, J.T.: Sex roles and achievement; in Christina, Landers, Psychology of motor behavior and sport, vol. 2 (Human Kinetics Publishers, Champaign 1977).

Jackson, D.N.; Ahmed, S.A.; Heapy, N.A.: Is achievement a unitary construct? J. Res. Per. *10:* 1–21 (1976).

Kagan, J.; Moss, H.P.: Birth to maturity (Wiley & Sons, New York 1962).

Kennicke, L.J.: Self profiles of highly skilled female athletes participating in two types of activities: structured and creative; MS, University Park (1972).

Maccoby, E.E.; Jacklin, C.N.: The psychology of sex differences (Stanford University Press, Stanford 1974).

Marmor, J.: Changing patterns of femininity: psychoanalytic implications; in Miller, Psychoanalysis and women (Brunner/Mazel, New York 1973).

Mehrabian, A: Measures of achieving tendency. Ed. Psy. Meas. *29:* 493–502 (1969).

Monk, S.V.: An investigation of the self and ideal self profiles and the dissonance between them among field hockey players; MS, University Park (1976).

Morgan, W.P.: Sport psychology; in Singer, The psychomotor domain: movement behavior (Lea & Febiger, Philadelphia 1972).

Snyder, E.E.; Kivlin, J.; Spreitzer, E.E.: Female athletes: an analysis of subjective and objective role conflict; in Landers, Harris, Christina, Proc. North American Society for the Psychology of Sport and Physical Activity (Pennsylvania State University, University Park 1975).

Spence, J.T.; Helmreich, R.L.: Masculinity and femininity: their psychological dimensions, correlates, and antecedents (University of Texas Press, Austin 1978).

Spence, J.T.; Helmreich, R.; Stapp, J.: Ratings of self and peers on sex-role attributes and their relation to self-esteem and conceptions of masculinity and femininity. J. Per. Soc. Psych. *32:* 29–39 (1975).

Weiner, B.; Freize, I.; Kukla, A.; Reed, L.; Rest, S.; Rosenbaum, R.M.: Perceiving the causes of success and failure (General Learning Press Module, New York 1971).

Prof. Dr. D.V. Harris, Center for Women and Sport, The Pennsylvania State University, University Park, PA 16802 (USA)

Medicine Sport, vol. 15, pp. 58–62 (Karger, Basel 1981)

Sugar and Spice and Everything Nice, Is that What Female Athletes Behave Like?

John H. Salmela

Département d'Education Physique, Université de Montreal, Montréal, Canada

> 'Frogs and snails and puppy dog tails.
> That's what little boys are made of.
> Sugar and spice and everything nice,
> That's what little girls are made of.'
> Traditional old English
> nursury rhyme

At a recent North American conference on the female athlete, *Harris* [1980] pointed out that greater gains of a social nature could be achieved by adopting the viewpoint that men and women are more alike than they are different. It was further pointed out that very early in life, boys and girls are socialized into traditional roles by reinforcing the expectancy that they are different, by such means as the above rhyme. *Harris* [1980] also contends that there is a lack of definitive data of a behavioral nature upon which to base a clear judgement on the nature of men and women in real sport situations.

This paper is an attempt to provide some behavioral evidence on men and women during the competitive moments at the Olympic Games. These data will be interpreted within the framework provided by *May* [1980] in which the concept of sexual androgyny is considered across a developmental dimension.

May [1980] presents convincing evidence, that goes against the prevailing orthodoxy on the psychology of women: that men and women differ significantly in terms of their psychological qualities as the result of the complex interweaving of biological disposition and cultural opportunism. However, these differences are unstable and tend to be magnified or reduced at different phases of the life span. Thus, for example, during the adolescent period the greatest gap in behavioral differences occurs and results in the demonstration of the archetypical behavior patterns that take on proportions that approach the level of parody.

Males typically press ahead, are anxious and irritable yet vulnerable and obsessed with decline, while females yield, show flexibility and respond caringly and willingly to social forces. With age, however, both sexes take on parts of themselves that they have underplayed at an earlier stage.

Having already demonstrated that they can adequately fulfill the stereotypic roles that society expects them to play, they adopt another set of behaviors that allows the emergence of previously suppressed dimensions. Thus, age interacts with various forms of behaviors within this androgynous view of human beings.

In the present study, the competitive behaviors of male and female gymnasts during the Montreal Olympic Games were observed using applied behavior analysis techniques. The sport of competitive gymnastics as the area of study would tend to minimize any sex-specific sport behaviors in that this activity is judged to be appropriate for both men and women. For both groups certain elements of power and strength must be included in a manner that results in beauty and virtuosity in the movement patterns. Thus, behaviors typical of male *machismo* observed in more violent sports would not bias the behavior differences between sexes.

Approximately one third (33.2%) of all gymnastic performances of 90.3% of the total population of gymnasts at the 1976 Olympic gymnastic competitions were observed by five trained observers. The average age of the male gymnasts was 23.8 years while that of the females was 18.0. The exact nature of the observational tool, the operational definitions, the statistical procedures, the inter-rater consensus and the supporting literature are reported fully elsewhere [*Salmela* et al., 1980].

Briefly, the results of this study can be summarized as follows: (1) that the women demonstrated a greater number of emotional behaviors than the men both prior to competing as well as a reaction to the quality of their performance and to the mark that it was awarded; (2) that the women spent significantly less time in social contact with their teammates during the 4 min prior to competing than did the men while being more often in the presence of their coach; (3) that the women received significantly less positive feedback from their teammates than did the men after having competed but received more from the coach; and (4) that these emotional and social behavioral patterns remained significantly different between the men and the women, but to varying degrees, independently of the society of origin of the gymnasts or the level of performance.

These results appear to depart from the currently espoused viewpoint on women in sport [*Harris*, 1980], that behavioral differences do not occur between the sexes. The present observations demonstrated reliable differences between the men and the women both during the pre- and post-competitive periods in a consistent manner for both the emotional and the social behaviors.

While the performance demands of the men's and women's disciplines are not identical, the fact that the precompetitive motor, instrumental and concentration behaviors of the men and women showed no differences, indicated that both groups prepared themselves somewhat similarly for the tasks at hand. It was only the incidence of emotional and ideo-motor behaviors that allowed the two sexes to be distinguished.

One essential condition that was not identical for populations of athletes was the respective ages of the two groups. As *May* [1980] points out, there is a likely interaction between the incidence of certain behaviors and the age of the individual. In the present case, assuming that both the groups of men and women began the sport at the same age, the men would have benefitted from about 5 more years of experience in the competitive arena as well as being further along on the biological timetable. Thus, most of the women in the present sample are either in or around the adolescent period, at which times behavioral profiles can be at their most extreme. The additional years of experience would have seasoned the men to the competitive stresses that occur at this level and perhaps provided them with more efficient coping strategies for stress management that then would translate to the behavioral level.

The social behaviors were also found to be reliably different for the men and women both prior to and after having competed. One explanation for this lack of social contact between the female teammates could be that their relative lack of competitive experience compared to the men would result in a narrowing of their attention and the tuning in to the immediate preparatory details that had to be considered and thus they had no additional capacity for the niceties of social contact with anyone else but the coach. An alternative explanation is that provided by *Bardwick* [1971]: that since women have not traditionally been socialized into the high achievement roles required for elite sport competition, they wore the cloak of competition with less ease. The perceived threat of their associates may have resulted in the exercising of subtle means of aggression towards their teammates, such as withholding of affection, in this case performance feedback, or by physically withdrawing from their presence.

Again, the effect of age and experience could magnify these differences in behavioral social patterns. The availability of a greater number of competitive experiences may have allowed the men the possibility of further streamlining their preparation procedures, thus freeing up some attentional capacity for social contacts with teammates. These age-related effects might also be such that a certain degree of competitive graciousness that is directed to one's teammates might evolve as the sport became placed within a broader perspective in life.

One might speculate that the males, being older, have already lived through similar anxiety-ridden competitive moments during their adolescence. Similarly, the women in the present situation appeared to be singularly preoccupied with the stresses inherent in this situation and could not afford the luxury of attending to the lot of their teammates. It is conceivable that once the women had additional competitive experiences, or merely by means of the aging process, these behavioral differences would be reduced to their baseline levels.

It appears to be quite clear that distinct androgynous tendencies surface when the behavioral patterns of elite male and female gymnasts are compared. The higher levels of emotional behavior and the detached social behaviors of the women resembled the profile of the assertive male. *Harris* [1980] has already dispelled the fallacies behind the arguments that sport masculinizes women, and it can now be seen as possibly a behavioral milepost in both male and female growth and development. What is unique in these data is that the males demonstrated a greater number of social behaviors to their teammates that could be interpreted as representing the yielding, caring female stereotype.

The resolution of this behavioral disparity appears to be within the concept of sexual androgyny; that both males and females possess the dimensions of assertiveness and yielding, instrumentality, and compassion, but to different degrees. In addition, the process of aging, with its potential for the integration of new coping strategies, may allow different emphases to be given to previously suppressed sets of behaviors. It seems that men and women in sport, as in other life activities, need no longer be held hostage to the traditional roles found in old nursury rhymes, but nor should they be to the prevailing orthodoxy of gender research.

References

Bardwick, J.: The psychology of women (Harper & Row, New York 1971).

Harris, D.V.: Psychological considerations of women in sports. Recorded cassette of North American Conf. on the Female Athlete (Simon Fraser University, Continuing Services, Burnaby 1980).

May, R.: Sex and fantasy: patterns of male and female development (Norton, New York 1980).

Salmela, J.H.; Petiot, B.; Hallé, M.; Règnier, G.: Competitive behaviors of olympic gymnasts (Thomas, Springfield 1980).

Dr. J. Salmela, Département d'Education Physique, Université de Montréal, Montréal, Que. (Canada)

Medicine Sport, vol. 15, pp. 63–66 (Karger, Basel 1981)

Differences in Athletic Aggression among Egyptian Female Athletes

M.H. Allawy

Faculty of Sports Education Helwan University, Cairo, Egypt

Introduction

Aggression, hostility and violence displayed in sport events are important issues facing contemporary sport. The control of such destructive behaviors which violate the sportsmanship, sport ethics and spirit of fair play may increase the value of sport to society. Additionally, such anti-social behavior expressed in sport competitions is sometimes reflected in spectator behavior and is likely to decrease the importance of sport status.

A variety of studies have investigated the relationship between aggressive behavior and indirect or vicarious participation, such as viewing various forms of physical activity [*Hartman*, 1969; *Turner*, 1970; *Goldstein and Arms*, 1971; *Leith*, 1978]. Other studies [*Husman*, 1955; *Volkamer*, 1972; *Lefebvre and Passer*, 1974; *Leith*, 1978; *Allawy*, 1978; *Soliman*, 1978] have investigated the relationship between aggressive behavior and direct participation in various forms of physical activity.

Leith [1978] reported that research concerning aggressive and vicarious or direct participation in physical activity is inconsistent and showed several contradictory results. He also pointed out some of the difficulties involved in arriving at a comprehensive definition of aggression in sport. This difficulty, in agreeing on a unitary definition, indicates the difficulty of trying to measure aggression in the sporting environment.

In this study athletic aggression is defined as any attempt to harm an opponent by physical, verbal or indirect means.

Purpose

This study was undertaken to determine if differences in athletic aggression (physical, verbal and indirect aggression) existed between Egyptian female athletes according to type of sport activity.

Procedure

90 Egyptian female superior athletes representing 3 groups of sport activities served as subjects for the investigation; they distributed as 30 athletes in each of the following groups: contact games (15 basketball and 15 handball players), non-contact games group (17 volleyball, 6 tennis, and 7 table tennis players), and individual sports group (13 track and field competitors and 17 swimmers).

All subjects were administered the Athletic Aggression Inventory [*Allawy*, 1978], which was developed to assess three different dimensions of athletic aggression:

Physical Aggression. Physical violence to harm an opponent, getting into fights with others, inflicting physical pain upon an opponent in order to achieve success, enjoy frustrating an opponent by physical means.

Verbal Aggression. Enjoy arguments with other competitors, threat and/or swear at others when something goes wrong during a contest, assault verbally an opponent in order to hurt her feelings.

Indirect Aggression. The opponent is not attacked directly but by devious means with the intent of hurting her.

The Athletic Aggression Inventory consisted of 27 statements, 9 statements for each of physical, verbal, and indirect aggression subscales, which were completed by each subject on a four-point scale.

Responses ranged from: strongly agree, agree, disagree to strongly disagree. No neutral middle scale was provided. Data were analyzed using row scores on each of the three subscales. The analysis of variance and the t-test for comparison of multiple means were used to treat the data.

Results

Significant differences were found among the subject groups in physical aggression ($F = 4.25$, $p < 0.5$) and in verbal aggression ($F = 3.65$, $p < 0.5$).

Subject groups did not significantly differ in indirect aggression (F = 1.87, p > 0.05).

To determine between which means difference existed the t-test technique was used. The results indicated that the contact games group scored significantly higher than the other two groups in physical aggression. The non-contact group and the individual sport group scored significantly higher than the contact games group in verbal aggression.

Discussion

These findings may support the hypothesis that physical and verbal aggression are related to the type of sport activity and that participants in different sport groups did not differ in indirect aggression.

The significant differences in physical and verbal aggression may in part be due to the nature of the sport activity. In face-to-face sport activity the opponent is attacked directly by getting into a fight with her. It may be considered that competition in contact games is full of frustrating situations which breed more physical aggression behavior than verbal aggression behavior. These findings are consistent with those of *Allawy* [1978] and *Soliman* [1978]. They found significant differences in physical and verbal aggression among athletes representing 12 different sports.

These findings are limited to the samples tested. Further research clearly determining whether there are differences in aggression dimensions among the various sport activities is required. The question of whether one group of female superior athletes is higher or lower in aggression dimensions than another female superior athletes group is important. For example, if we find that one group of female superior athletes is higher in physical aggression, additional research may reveal that it is the participation in such a form of sport activity that causes higher physical aggression. Or it may be that only those personalities with initially higher aggression traits are able to succeed in this form of sport activity. Or it may be that there is a reciprocal cause-and-effect relationship between these two factors. Further studies on athletic aggression could investigate if there are carry-over effects.

Berkowitz [1962], in discussing the effect of competitive sports on aggression, pointed out that aggressive sports probably do not eliminate aggressive habits. The present author suggests that in future research on aggression in sport more attention to the problem of state-and-trait aggressiveness should be considered.

Summary

90 Egyptian female athletes representing 3 groups of sport activities were administered the Athletic Aggression Inventory. Differences between research samples were
examined with Anova. Results of statistical analyses indicated significant differences in
physical and verbal aggression among the various groups of female athletes (contact,
non-contact games, and individual sports). Subjects did not significantly differ in indirect
aggression. It was concluded that the question of whether one group of female athletes
is higher or lower in athletic aggression dimensions than another female athletes group
is important.

References

Allawy, M.: Sports psychology; 4th ed., pp. 230–262 (Dar El-Maarif, Cairo 1978).
Berkowitz, L.: Aggression, a social psychological analysis, p. 205 (McGraw-Hill, New
    York 1962).
Goldstein, J.; Arms, R.: Effects of observing athletic contests on hostility. Sociometry
    34: 83–90 (1971).
Hartman, D.: Influence of symbolically modelled instrumental aggression and pain cues on
    aggressive behavior. J. Pers. Soc. Psy. 11: 280–288 (1969).
Husman, B.: Aggression in boxers and wrestlers as measured by projective techniques.
    Res. Quart. 26: 421–425 (1955).
Lefebvre, L.; Passer, M.: The effect of game location and importance on aggression in
    team sport. Int. J. Sp. Psy. 5: 102–110 (1974).
Leith, L.: The psychological assessment of aggression in sport; in Simri, Proc. Int. Symp.
    on Psychological Assessment in Sport, pp. 126–135 (Netanya 1978).
Soliman, I.: Aggression among Egyptian athletes and its relationship with some selected
    variables. Unpublished Ph. D. Diss., Cairo (1978).
Turner, E.: The effect of viewing college football, basketball, and wrestling, on the elicited
    aggressive responses of male spectators; in Kenyon, Contemporary psychology of
    sport, pp. 325–328 (Athletic Institute, Chicago 1970).
Volkamer, N.: Investigations into the aggressiveness in competitive social systems. Sport-
    wissenschaft 1: 33–64 (1972).

Prof. Dr. Mohamed H.Allawy, 62 Abasia Street, Cairo (Egypt)

Medicine Sport, vol. 15, pp. 67–73 (Karger, Basel 1981)

Machover Test Applied to 130 Italian Female Top Athletes

S. Rota, E. Baldo, M. Benzi, S. Federici

Istituto di Medicina dello Sport, Roma, Italia

Introduction and Purpose

The Machover test is a projective technique, and as such, it gives some information about the personality of the person taking the test.

There is a fundamental concept for the drawing techniques, involving personality which does not develop in a vacuum but in the movement, feelings and thoughts of an individual. In general, as *Machover* [1949] stated, 'a drawing of a person is an expression of self, of the body, in its environment'. What is put on the paper can be characterized as 'an image of the body', it can be considered as a complex reflection of self-esteem, a self-image.

The basis for the interpretation of Machover's test is the concept that the subject will draw a projection of the image she/he has of her/his own body, i.e. a projection of self.

The self-image that each individual has of himself or herself evolves in time; it is the end result of experience, identification, projections, and introjections. It follows that the composed image, which is the drawn figure, is intimately united to the self in all of its ramifications. We chose the Machover test to analyse the way athletic women perceive themselves and their bodies.

Procedure

We studied 130 female athletes using the Machover test; they have trained in 13 different sports on a national level and their average age was 19.3 years (table I).

The instructions for the test were as follows: draw a complete human figure, from head to toes, emphasizing that it was not a test of their ability to draw. Once the drawing was completed, they received a second piece of paper with the instructions to draw another human figure of the opposite sex of the first. Thus, we obtained two drawings: a male figure and a female figure.

In our analysis we gave particular attention to the drawing of the female figure; the following elements, in that order, were considered: the succession of the figures; size and location of the figure on the paper; the position: front, profile, back; expression: smiling, aggressive, sad; characteristics: ornate, bare, stylized; examination of the hands: hidden, clenched; distortions and omissions.

Results and Discussion

The first item, as table II illustrates, was the succession of the figures, which sex was drawn first. In the researches of *Abt and Bellak* [1967] with 5,000 subjects, the first figure drawn by 87% of them corresponded to their own sex. This study and numerous other research confirm the fact that usually the first figure drawn is that of the same sex of the person making the drawing, seldom is it the opposite sex. In our study the percent of women athletes whose first figure was their same sex was significantly lower (55.4%) compared to a sampling of the average population.

Why do many athletic women draw first a figure of a person of the opposite sex? There can be many answers to this question, the fact remains that when someone is asked 'to draw a person' she/he must solve various problems and difficulties looking for a close model. In the present day athletic world, it is easy for the woman athlete to be surrounded by male figures (technicians, directors, coaches, champions, etc.) who, generally, are her reference models.

We also want to point out that there was a significantly different distribution of those whose first figure was a person of the opposite sex among the various sports included in our research. The highest percent of male drawings first (70%) was by those who play volleyball and play football, and the lowest percent was by those who practiced artistic gymnastics and skating (20%).

The size of the drawn figures was for the most part (78.46%) average. The majority (84.62%) placed their figures in the centre of the paper, which seems to indicate a good capacity to adjust to their environment and good harmony with their bodies.

Most of the drawings were the front position (83%) which indicated their availability and readiness to relate with the external world.

Table I. Machover test: examined sample

Sport	n	Mean age, years: months
Archery	10	21:6
Basketball	10	22:7
Canoeing	10	20
Fencing	10	22
Football	10	22:6
Gymnastics	10	15:5
Handball	10	19:1
Skating	10	17
Skiing	10	18
Swimming	10	15
Tennis	10	15:9
Track and field	10	21:7
Volleyball	10	20:7
Total	130	19:36

Table II. Machover test: structural aspects

	n	%
First figure		
Woman	72	55.4
Man	58	44.6
Size		
Small	15	11.54
Medium	102	78.46
Large	13	10
Space placing		
Left side	6	4.61
Right side	2	1.53
Top side	10	7.69
Bottom side	2	1.53
Centre	110	84.62
Position		
Front view	108	83
Side view	18	13.8
Back view	2	1.53
Other	2	1.53

Table III. Machover test: formal aspects

	n	%
Figure		
Stylized	10	7.69
Ornate	23	17.69
Bare	9	6.92
Hands		
Hidden		
Both	26	20
One	7	5.38
Fists	9	6.92
Facial Expression		
Smiling	45	34.61
Aggressive	12	9.23
Sad	21	16.15
None	8	6.15
Other	44	33.84
Movement	10	7.69

Formal Aspects (table III)

Analysing the way the athletes drew the figure of their own sex we found that 7.69% drew a stylized figure. According to Machover this is typical of those who place more importance on their own needs.

The clothing represents the way the person apparently is or wants to appear to others. The particular care in drawing the clothing, present in 17.69% of the athletes, might indicate an adaptation to a socially traditional aspect, or it might be an expression of narcissism through the clothing.

The nude drawing (6.92%) could be a challenge to social standards or it could be an expression of the presence of sexual conflicts.

The hands are manipulatory organs, organs of contact: they act, establish relations, punish or defend. In 25.38% of the drawings of the subject's own sex, the hands were hidden: this could indicate difficulty in making contact with one's environment and/or the presence of guilt feelings related to manipulatory activity. The clenched fists in 6.92% of the drawings indicate repressed aggression.

The expression on the drawn face usually gives information about how the subject feels. In our study 34.61% of the athletes drew the figure of their own sex with a smiling face; 16.15% projected a sad image of self; and

Table IV. Machover test: distortions and omissions

Body part	Distortions		Omissions	
	n	%	n	%
Body	3	2.3	0	0
Head	14	10.76	0	0
Hair	0	0	1	0.76
Face	1	0.76	3	2.3
Eyes	0	0	5	3.84
Pupils	0	0	7	5.38
Nose	0	0	3	2.3
Mouth	2	1.53	5	3.84
Neck	1	0.76	0	0
Bust	1	0.76	0	0
Arms				
Both	7	5.38	0	0
One	0	0	1	0.76
Hands				
Both	4	3.07	15	11.53
One	0	0	4	3.07
Legs				
Both	9	6.92	2	1.53
One	0	0	2	1.53
Feet	3	2.3	12	9.23
Total	45		60	

9.23% had an aggressive expression. Hence, the majority of these athletes have a 'happy' relationship with their own image.

Movement is a characteristic that is seldom found in the drawings of the Machover test; it was present in 7.69% of the drawings by our athletes. A moving figure is related to interior creativity, an indication of good psychic dynamism.

Distortions (table IV)

The parts of the body that were more frequently out of proportion were: the head (14 cases = 10.76%), the legs (9 cases = 6.92%) and the arms (7 cases = 5.38%).

In all 14 cases the head was too large in proportion to the rest of the body; most of these drawings were made by athletes who practice gymnastics (3 cases) and swimming (3 cases). This seems to indicate an underevaluation of the body compared to the head or the mind. The sports with the larger number of athletes drawing distorted figures were: gymnastics (6 cases), track and field, skiing, swimming, and football (5 cases each). The sports with the least number of athletes drawing distorted figures were: basketball (none), volleyball, canoeing, and archery (1 case each).

These data, which might be interpreted as a measure of the awareness the athletes have of their body scheme, were rather surprising, particularly for the gymnasts. However, the young age of these athletes must be kept in mind (15.6 years); after swimming it was the lowest average age of the various groups of athletes we studied. On the other hand, the average age of the athletes whose drawings were more proportionate – the basketball players – was the highest, i.e. 22.8 years.

Omissions (table IV)

According to *Machover* [1949] the omission of an important part of the body indicates the presence of internal, unconscious conflicts related to the omitted part.

The more significant omissions are: the hands (14.60%, of this 11.53% omitted both hands and 3.07% one hand), the feet (9.23%), and the pupils (5.38%). These parts of the body give information about the way the subject contacts external reality. Hence, their omission could indicate difficulty in relating with the external world.

The omission of the pupils, more frequent among the tennis players (2.3%), might indicate a possible withdrawal in self. It seems coherent that individuals who refuse to see reality objectively, might omit the pupils.

Furthermore, *Machover* [1949] suggests that the feet also have a certain sexual symbolism and their omission could indicate some sexual conflict.

Conclusions

The profile of the high-level women athlete – the conclusion of our research with 130 female athletes – shows a sufficiently good identification with her role. This is concluded from the fact that most of the athletes drew a figure of their own sex first, and the figures have a smiling expression. Awareness of the corporal scheme (concluded from the lack of proportion in the figures) seemed to depend more on age than on the type of sport practiced. Some of the athletes we studied have internal conflicts (concluded from the omissions in their drawings).

It is our intention to extend our research to a group – comparable in number and average age – of women who are not intensively involved in sport activity.

Summary

The Machover Draw-a-Person Test (DAP) is a psychodiagnostic projective test in order to point out the basic attitudes of an individual towards his (or her) own body and self-esteem. This test was administered to 130 top female Italian athletes. The authors report the results of their research showing the differences in the drawings among the participants of different sport activities.

References

Abt, L.; Bellak, L.: La psicologia proiettiva (Longanesi, Milano 1967).
Machover, K.: Personality projection in the drawing of the human figure (Thomas, Springfield 1949).

Dr. Sergio Rota, Via G. Pepe 37, I-00185 Roma (Italy)

Kinanthropometry

Medicine Sport, vol. 15, pp. 74–89 (Karger, Basel 1981)

Proportionality and Body Composition in Male and Female Olympic Athletes: A Kinanthropometric Overview

W.D. Ross, R.M. Leahy, D.T. Drinkwater, P.L. Swenson

Department of Kinesiology, Simon Fraser University, Burnaby, Canada

Kinanthropometry is a scientific specialization which is in the process of identifying itself. As outlined in figure 1, the research enterprise has been delimited to establish bounds wherein rigorous methodology can be developed; yet, it is sufficiently comprehensive to incorporate research workers and professionals representing many disciplines and affiliations.

We shall not attempt a general introduction but restrict our presentation to a discourse on proportionality and body composition of male and female Olympic athletes using a unisex reference human as a metaphorical calculation device.

Of course, being in Italy, any mention of human proportionality evokes the awesome historical presence of *Leonardo da Vinci*. If he were able to span the some 460 years after his death, it might amuse him to learn his

IDENTIFICATION	SPECIFICATION	APPLICATION	RELEVANCE
Kinanthropometry	For the study of human	to help understand	with implications for
MOVEMENT	SIZE	GROWTH	MEDICINE
HUMAN	SHAPE	EXERCISE	EDUCATION
MEASUREMENT	PROPORTION	PERFORMANCE	GOVERNMENT
	COMPOSITION	NUTRITION	with respect for individual rights in the service of humankind
	MATURATION		
	GROSS FUNCTION		

Fig. 1. Kinanthropometry: 'an emerging scientific specialization'.

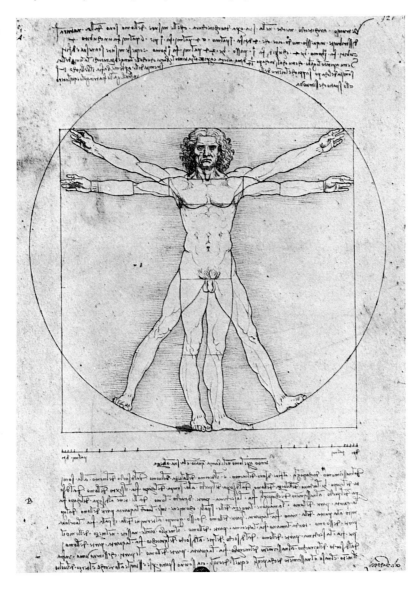

Fig. 2. Leonardo da Vinci: Vitruvian Man.

Vitruvian Man illustrating proportional characteristics of the adult male has become a symbol for the universality of humankind. Admittedly, as shown in figure 2, his drawing does have a sense of harmony, a feeling of omnipotence, and it does command attention. Yet, one wonders how a drawing of a middle-aged, Caucasian male is an appropriate symbol. If we were to establish a universal prototype, surely it would be more feminine than masculine, under 18 years of age, multi-racial and, probably, tea-coloured.

The Phantom

Our approach to the study of human proportionality was to establish a unisex reference human or *phantom*. Male and female data gleaned from the literature was geometrically adjusted to a standard stature (5 feet 7 inches, 170.18 cm) and over 100 anthropometric measures (p) and their standard deviations (s) have been specified [*Ross and Wilson*, 1974; *Eiben* et al., 1976; *Hebbelinck and Borms*, 1978; *Drinkwater and Ross*, 1980; *Skibinska*, 1979].

The stratagem essentially consists of expressing differences from the *phantom* as z-values calculated by the following general formula:

$$z = \frac{1}{s} \left[v \left(\frac{170.18}{h} \right)^d - p \right], \tag{1}$$

where z is a proportionality score, z-value; s is the phantom standard deviation for variable (v); v is any given variable; 170.18 is the phantom stature constant; h is the subject's obtained height; d is a dimensional exponent where in the geometrical scaling procedure all lengths, breadths, girths and skinfold thicknesses $d = 1$; all areas $d = 2$; all masses and volumes $d = 3$; p is the given phantom value for variable (v).

A z-value of 0.0 for a given variable indicates that the subject has the same proportion as the phantom. A positive z-value indicates that the subject is proportionaly larger than the phantom for the given variable, whereas a negative value indicates that the subject is proportionally smaller. The use of the stratagem has been demonstrated in studies of athletes by *Hebbelinck and Ross* [1974], *Ross and Wilson* [1974], *Ross* [1976], *Eiben* et al. [1976], *Skibinska* [1979], *Ross* et al. [1980], and *Hebbelinck* et al. [1980]. It has also been used in secular trend studies by *Vajda and Hebbelinck* [1978] and *Eiben* [1978]; in cross-sectional studies of boys and girls by *Hebbelinck and Borms* [1978]; in longitudinal growth studies by *Ross* [1978] and *Ross* et al. [1980] and in studies of sex chromosomal aneuploidy by *Eiben* [1980], *Miller* et al. [1980] and *Bosze* et al. [1980].

Fractionation Tactic

In keeping with the pioneering work of *Matiegka* [1921] and *Perkal* [1953] an application of the phantom stratagem was found for the anthropometric fractionation of body mass as discussed by *Drinkwater and Ross* [1980]. Rejecting a patently false assumption of a constant density of the non-fat component which is essential to the conventional 2-component models for assessing body composition, the new tactic assumes the body can be fractionated into *four components* which can be derived independently of obtained total body mass by use of phantom z-values. As reported in the original paper, the sum of fractionated fat, bone, muscle and residual masses by this procedure accounted for total body mass in men and women ($n = 939$, $r = 0.97$, difference of mean 0.3% of obtained values).

Theoretically, any anthropometric indicator of a particular tissue mass should deviate as the mass of that tissue. For example, if skinfold thicknesses are used to indicate the fat mass, a mean deviation of -1.0 z for the skinfolds of a given subject would be related to a mean deviation of the fat mass of -1.0 z. Since the specified phantom fat mass (p) is 12.13 kg and its standard deviation (s) is 3.25 kg, the derived fat mass would be the difference, 12.31–3.25 or 8.88 kg. This would then have to be rescaled to the subject's actual stature by dividing 8.88 by $(170.18/h)^3$.

Thus, the general formula for obtaining fat, muscle, bone and residual masses is as follows:

$$M = \frac{\bar{Z} \times S + P}{\left(\dfrac{170.18}{h}\right)^3}. \tag{2}$$

M is the mass fractionation, e.g. fat, muscle, bone or residual. $\bar{Z}$ is the *mean* for measures selected to indicate the fraction calculated from p and s values shown in table I (i.e. skinfolds to yield fat mass; bone breadths to yield bone mass; girths over muscular parts corrected by skinfold thicknesses to yield muscle mass; and torso measures to yield residual mass). s is the phantom standard deviation for fractionated fat, bone, muscle and residual masses shown in table I. p is the given phantom values for fat, bone, muscle and residual masses shown in table I. 170.18 is the phantom stature constant. h is the subject's stature or height. 3 is a dimensional exponent relating linear measures to volume and mass.

Subjects

The fractionation tactic was evoked to view proportionality and body composition characteristics of male and female Olympic athletes in four sports and a reference sample

Table I. Phantom specifications for estimation of fractionated body mass

Mass	Subset indicators	p	s
Fat, kg		12.13	3.25
	triceps skinfold, mm	15.4	4.47
	subscapular skinfold	17.2	5.07
	suprailiac skinfold[1]	15.4	4.47
	abdominal skinfold	25.4	7.78
	front thigh skinfold	27.0	8.33
	medial calf skinfold	16.0	4.67
Bone, kg		10.49	1.57
	bi-epicondylar humerus width, cm	6.48	0.35
	bi-epicondylar femur width	9.52	0.48
	wrist girth (distal to styloids)	16.35	0.72
	ankle girth (smallest)	21.71	1.33
Muscle, kg		25.55	2.99
	relaxed arm girth − π triceps sf, cm	22.05	1.91
	chest girth − π subscapular sf	82.36	4.86
	thigh girth − π front thigh sf	47.34	3.59
	calf girth − π medial calf sf	30.22	1.97
	forearm girth[1]	25.13	1.41
Residual, kg		16.41	1.90
	biacromial breadth, cm	38.04	1.92
	transverse chest width	27.92	1.74
	bi-iliocristal breadth	28.84	1.75
	anterior-posterior chest depth	17.50	1.38

Skinfold correction $= (\pi \times sf)/10$.
Bi-iliocristal breadth substituted for ankle girth for bone mass determination in this study.
[1] Optional inclusion.

of university students. The subjects classified as runners and swimmers were drawn from different events and are not specific types as were the gymnasts and rowers. In order to provide a non-sport control, a sample of men and women university students from three British Columbia, Canada, universities were recruited for the purpose. The students were volunteers from a general education exercise class, a non-specialist teacher training class in physical education, and a student residence. The sample was arbitrary and possibly more disposed toward exercise than the general university population.

Methods

All data was collected by anthropometrists involved in the Montreal Olympic Games Anthropological Project (MOGAP) using techniques reported by *de Garay* et al. [1974] amplified as discussed by *Borms* et al. [1977].

Table II. Anthropometric fraction of body mass of male and female Olympic athletes and university students

Mass	Runners		Gymnasts		Swimmers		Rowers		Students	
	m (25) f (20)		m (11) f (15)		m (33) f (32)		m (66) f (51)		m (152) f (94)	
Fat										
Z	-2.41	-1.81	-2.37	-1.73	-2.00	-0.94	-2.04	-1.07	-1.61	-0.29
SE	0.03	0.06	0.09	0.09	0.05	0.09	0.04	0.08	0.06	0.10
Kg	4.75	5.81	4.38	5.57	6.49	8.60	7.80	9.36	7.92	10.38
SD	0.80	1.14	1.11	1.02	2.81	1.91	1.56	2.24	2.76	2.98
%	7.21	10.92	6.90	10.92	8.82	14.88	8.78	14.24	10.96	18.04
Bone										
Z	-0.40	-1.32	0.98	-0.18	0.29	-0.56	0.31	-0.66	0.06	-0.63
SE	0.12	0.16	0.20	0.19	0.13	0.12	0.09	0.10	0.06	0.08
Kg	10.90	7.81	11.85	8.74	12.68	9.09	15.52	10.15	12.20	8.76
SD	1.45	1.23	1.11	1.25	1.73	1.31	1.43	1.19	1.58	1.20
%	16.54	14.67	18.67	13.13	19.24	15.73	17.48	15.44	16.88	15.22
Muscle										
Z	1.18	0.71	1.81	0.75	1.55	0.53	1.47	0.77	1.24	0.32
SE	0.13	0.12	0.15	0.10	0.13	0.09	0.07	0.08	0.06	0.08
Kg	32.08	25.69	30.54	23.82	3.98	25.66	42.43	29.93	33.78	24.48
SD	3.48	2.95	2.64	2.63	4.19	2.75	2.83	2.08	3.93	2.64
%	48.67	48.27	48.12	46.70	47.55	44.40	47.78	45.53	46.75	42.19
Residual										
Z	-0.47	-0.76	0.03	-0.72	0.19	-0.20	-0.08	-0.65	-0.26	-0.71
SE	0.10	0.16	0.09	0.18	0.61	0.09	0.07	0.08	-0.05	0.06
Kg	11.11	13.09	16.26	12.88	19.43	15.19	23.06	16.30	18.36	13.92
SD	1.63	2.04	1.61	1.57	2.06	1.82	1.87	1.30	2.03	1.50
%	26.00	24.60	25.62	25.32	26.41	26.28	25.97	24.79	25.41	24.19
Predicted	65.92	54.62	63.46	51.01	73.57	57.79	88.81	65.74	72.26	57.54
Obtained	64.85	53.22	63.02	50.86	72.98	58.53	89.68	67.36	72.35	57.48
% Difference 100 (P-O)/O	-1.42	-2.59	-0.48	0.46	0.94	-1.42	-0.97	-2.40	0.01	0.21

Analysis

For each of the ten samples, fractionated values are shown in table II. The z-value and its standard error which is the standard deviation of z divided by the square root of the number in the sample gives an indication of the sample proportional fractional body mass. The calculated fractional masses in kilograms and the standard deviations are the predicted body composition values for the particular sample. These fractionations are also shown as percent values of the predicted total body mass. Thus, their sum will equal 100 for each sample. At the bottom of table II, the predicted and obtained total body mass values are shown. The percent difference shows how closely the predicted values account for the total body mass. All of the percent differences shown are trivial since body mass itself is not invariable but reflects daily variation as well as possible acute training effects in the athletic samples.

It is beyond the scope of our introductory paper to discuss all of the summarized information. One of the advantages of standard scores or z-values is that they invite comparison. The 40 z-values yield 780 possible comparisons. Only some of these are realistic. These might include 60 comparisons of masses within each subgroup, 20 comparisons of like masses between males and females within the same event and 80 comparisons of the same mass within the same sex.

Rather than use unwieldly statistical analysis in meaningless comparisons, our approach is to use an inspectional procedure which permits the investigator to make any particular comparison he or she feels is pertinent. As an ancillary demonstration we plotted mean z-values plus and minus two standard error distances on transparent acetate sheets for each fractional mass, for each of the ten samples. This was done by computer on a flat-bed plotter since we wished to produce sheets in quantity for distribution at this presentation. However, simple hand plotting would be adequate for most instances.

To illustrate the procedure, we compared male and female gymnasts with their same sex norms in figures 3 and 4, and with each other in figure 5. As shown in figure 3, the male gymnasts had proportionally smaller fat mass but greater bone and muscle mass than the male norms. As shown in figure 4, the female gymnasts had smaller fat mass and greater muscle mass than the female norms. They were not, however, larger in bone mass. Neither gymnastic groups were significantly different than their same sex counterpart in residual mass.

As shown in figure 5, the sexual dimorphism between male and female gymnasts was apparent for each fractional mass with the males having less fat and greater bone, muscle and residual proportional masses than the females. The marked disposition to lightness in female gymnasts reflects the ascendency of the small, late-maturing girl gymnast who apparently has the necessary structural requirements for the sport. The male gymnast, on the other hand, apparently has an advantage from his late adolescent spurt in muscular skeletal robustness which generally follows peak height velocity

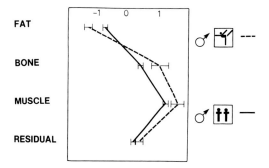

Fig. 3. Female Olympic gymnasts and university students.

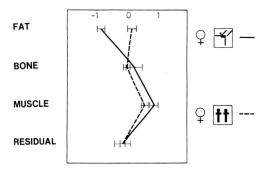

Fig. 4. Male Olympic gymnasts and university students.

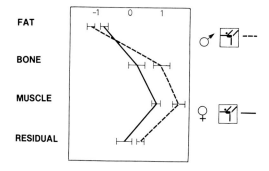

Fig. 5. Male and female Olympic gymnasts.

and, in growing boys, may be as late as 19 or 20 years of age. The implications for selectivity and training for the characteristic structural differences in male and female gymnasts are well-known.

Proportionality and body composition are only two aspects in the complex appraisal and guidance process in sport. Our 4-component model has some conceptual and interpretative advantages over the 2-component model. At best, we claim our confusion is only at a slightly higher level when we do not have to assume a constant density of the non-fat mass. We do not have final answers. The blatant assumption we share with other methods that there is a simple relationship between fat mass and skinfold thickness is vulnerable to challenges. Indeed, we already have cadaver dissection data from a joint venture with Dr. *Jan Clarys* of the Vrije Universiteit Brussel which we expect will soon force us to modify our 4-component model in that we shall not be able to derive fat directly from skinfolds or use unweighted z-values to apportion each fractional mass in divergent subjects. Our present method, or any method for that matter, is only a partial answer to the problem of quantification of human body composition. Thus, in the advance of our area, we must not be dismayed. It is the nature of science to build new edifices from the building blocks salvaged from ruined structures.

We have a splendid gathering of scientists from the international research community at this important congress in historic Rome. Our hosts well understand that scientific advance in important matters, such as women in sport, comes from the crucible of human interaction and determinative discussion. All of us have areas of ignorance and insight. We can learn and teach one another as friends and colleagues.

While it is essential to be charitable to all scientific propositions, each of us should exercise discretion and give attention to rigour in our reports. We might leave it to new Doctors of Philosophy to remind us of the holy writ of method, experimental design, statistical tests, and probability statements. We welcome them and encourage them to learn and contribute.

We should also apply four other criteria for evaluating our tactic, or any other scientific proposition. (1) Does it permit one to predict? (2) Does it link facts to the empirical phenomena observed? (3) Does it lead to new inferences? (4) Does it have practical value in the conduct of human affairs?

This congress is a bold attempt, at a time of political unrest, to focus world scientific attention on women in sport. It is appropriate that kinanthropometry has been designated as a thematic area. It cannot be excluded, for this area is the quantitative link between human structure and function and must be regarded as a basic and indispensible scientific enterprise.

Summary

Kinanthropometry as an emerging scientific specialization was viewed in terms of body composition using a unisex reference human or phantom to estimate fat, bone, muscle and residual masses. When this tactic was applied to data obtained on male and female Montreal Olympic runners, gymnasts, swimmers, rowers and university students, the sum of the fractionated masses accounted for all but 0.01–2.59% of the obtained body mass. The tactic was viewed in the context of kinanthropometry and the need for scientific advance in the area of in vivo human body composition assessment.

Acknowledgements

The data assembled in this paper were from MOGAP (Montreal Olympic Games Anthropological Project) with basic funding through the Université de Montréal by the Government of Quebec (Haut-Commissariat à la Jeunesse, aux Loisirs et aux Sports) with substantial support of the following sources: Vrije Universiteit Brussel; National Fund for Scientific Research (NFWO), Belgium; San Diego State College Foundation; Simon Fraser University President's Research Grant, and Simon Fraser University Operational Grant for Kinanthropometric Research, Canada Research Council (A9402). The authors recognize the contribution of colleagues from the University of Texas, Université de Montréal, Université Laval, the University of Western Ontario, San Diego State University and the Vrije Universiteit Brussel. Furthermore, the authors acknowledge the contribution of MOGAP anthropometrists and colleagues *Andree Vajda-Janyk* and *R.A. Faulkner* and the collaboration of Dr. *Bruce Howe*, University of Victoria, and Dr. *S.A. Brown*, University of British Columbia, in the assembly of control data.

References

Borms, J.; Hebbelinck, M.; Carter, J.E.L.; Ross, W.D.; Yuhasz, M.S.; Lariviere, G.: Standardization of basic anthropometry in Olympic athletes – the MOGAP procedure; in Novotny, Titlbachova, Methods of Functional Anthropology, Prague 1977, pp. 31–39 (Universitas Carolina, Prague 1979).

Bosze, P.; Eiben, O.G.; Gaal, M.; Laszlo, J.: Body measurements of patients with streak gonads and their bearing on the karyotype. Hum. Genet. *54:* 355–360 (1980).

Drinkwater, D.T.; Ross, W.D.: Anthropometric fractionation of body mass; in Ostyn, Beunen, Simons, Kinanthropometry, vol. II, pp. 177–188 (University Park Press, Baltimore 1980).

Eiben, O.G.: Changes in body measures and proportions in children based on Komend Growth Study; in Gedda, Parisi, Auxology: human growth in health and disorder, pp. 187–198 (Academic Press, London 1978).

Eiben, O.G.; Ross, W.D.; Christensen, W.; Faulkner, R.H.: Proportionality characteristics of female athletes. Antrop. Kozl. *20:* 55–67 (1976).

Eiben, O.G.: Recent data on variability in physique: some aspects of proportionality; in Ostyn, Beunen, Simons, Kinanthropometry, vol. II, pp. 69–77 (University Park Press, Baltimore 1980).

Garay, A.L. de; Levine, L.; Carter, J.E.L.: Genetic and anthropological studies of Olympic athletes (Academic Press, New York 1974).

Hebbelinck, M.; Borms, J.: Körperliches Wachstum und Leistungsfähigkeit bei Schulkindern, Sportmedizinische Schriftenreihe 15 (Barth, Leipzig 1978).

Hebbelinck, M.; Ross, W.D.: Kinanthropometry and biomechanics; in Nelson, Morehouse, Biomechanics. IV. Science and Medicine in Sport, vol. 9, pp. 537–552 (University Park Press, Baltimore 1974).

Hebbelinck, M.; Ross, W.D.; Carter, J.E.L.; Borms, J.: Anthropometric characteristics of female Olympic rowers. Can. J. appl. Sport. Sci. 5: 255–262 (1980).

Matiegka, J.: The testing of physical fitness. Am. J. phys. Anthrop. 4: 223–230 (1921).

Miller, R.; Ross, W.D.; Roede, M.: Sex chromosome aneuploidy and anthropometry: a new proportionality assessment using the phantom stratagem. Am. J. med. Genet. 5: 125–135 (1980).

Perkal, J.: Owskaznikkach Antropologicznych. Prezegl. Antropol. Poznan 19 (1953). Also in Perkal, J.; Szczotka, F.: Eine neue Methode der Analyse eines Kollektivs von Merkmalen. Biom. Z. 2: 108–116 (1960).

Ross, W.D.: Metaphorical models for the study of human shape and proportionality; in Broekhoff, Physical education sports and the sciences, pp. 284–304 (Microform Publications, University of Oregon, Eugene 1976).

Ross, W.D.: Kinanthropometry: an emerging scientific specialization; in Landry, Orban, Biomechanics of sport and kinanthropometry, vol. 6, pp. 269–288 (Symposia Specialists, Miami 1978).

Ross, W.D.; Drinkwater, D.T.; Bailey, D.A.; Marshall, G.W.; Leahy, R.M.: Kinanthropometry: traditions and new perspectives; in Ostyn, Beunen, Simons, Kinanthropometry, vol. II, pp. 3–27 (University Park Press, Baltimore 1980).

Ross, W.D.; Wilson, N.C.: A stratagem for proportional growth assessment; in Borms, Hebbelinck, Children and exercise. Acta paediat. belg. 28: suppl., pp. 169–183 (1974).

Skibinska, A.: Antropometryczny model czlowieka. Wychowanie Fizyczne i Sport 4: 3–11 (1979).

Vajda, A.; Hebbelinck, M.: Secular growth trend data in Belgian population since 1840; in Borms, Hebbelinck, Pediatric work physiology. Medicine Sport, vol. 11, pp. 134–139 (Karger, Basel 1978).

Dr. W.D. Ross, Department of Kinesiology, Simon Fraser University, Burnaby, B.C. V5A 1S6 (Canada)

Medicine Sport, vol. 15, pp. 85–116 (Karger, Basel 1981)

Somatotypes of Female Athletes

J.E. Lindsay Carter

Department of Physical Education, San Diego State University, San Diego, Calif., USA

Introduction

The morphological characteristics of athletes are of interest to the sports scientist and kinanthropometrist, for competitive sport demands the utmost from the body and it is therefore reasonable to expect to find in athletes demonstration of the relationship of structure and function [*Carter*, 1970]. One method of describing human morphology is through somatotyping, which is a classification of total body form and shape expressed as a simple rating on continuous scales. The usefulness of somatotyping for describing athletes from different sports has been demonstrated in studies such as those by *Tanner* [1964], *Carter* [1970], *de Garay* et al. [1974], and *Stepnicka* [1977]. In a summary of the contributions of somatotyping to kinanthropometry, *Carter* [1980a] pointed out differences among populations and between sexes, and relationships with maturation, body composition, and physical performance. From these and other studies we find that there is much more information on male than on female athletes. The first review of the somatotypes of female athletes was made by *Carter* [1970], and the samples consisted of 5 sports groups, two samples of dancers and two of physical education majors. During the past decade increased interest in female athletes has resulted in a number of studies using somatotyping but no adequate synthesis has been made of the available material.

The purpose of this paper is to review present knowledge of, and provide new information on, the somatotypes of female athletes. Special emphasis is placed on age, sport and event, level of competition, and sexual dimorphism. Additional knowledge of the body structure of successful female athletes in different sports can lead to a better understanding of the elements needed for optimal performance, and improved methods of selection and training.

Methods

The somatotype is a quantitative description of the present morphological conformation and composition of the body. It is expressed in a three-number rating that describes the body as a whole and is a rating of what the body looks like. The rating represents the evaluation of three components (endomorphy, mesomorphy, and ectomorphy) of the physique. Endomorphy refers to the relative fatness of the physique; mesomorphy refers to the musculo-skeletal development per unit of height; and ectomorphy refers to the relative linearity of the physique [*Carter*, 1980b]. The Heath-Carter somatotype method is adaptable for use in rating both sexes of all ages, and is a rating of the present somatotype; no assumptions are made regarding permanence of the somatotype. This method is appropriate for studies in kinanthropometry [*Carter and Heath*, 1971]. The studies reported in this paper used the somatotype method of *Heath and Carter* [1967]. The subjects were rated by the anthropometric method in 90% of the samples, the photoscopic method, or the anthropometric plus photoscopic method [*Carter*, 1980b; *Heath and Carter*, 1967]. For some samples the mean somatotype was estimated from means of anthropometric variables used in calculation of individual anthropometric somatotypes. The estimated mean is usually within 0.1 of the mean calculated from individual somatotypes.

Means and standard deviations for the following variables (where available) for each sample are presented in the tables: age, height, weight, height/cube root of weight, endomorphy, mesomorphy, and ectomorphy. In table I the somatotype dispersion index and somatotype attitudinal mean are also shown. The somatotype dispersion index (SDI) is the mean of the distances of each somatotype from the mean somatotype as plotted on the somatochart and are in the Y-units of the X, Y coordinates of the two-dimensional plot [*Ross and Wilson*, 1973]. The somatotype attitudinal mean (SAM) is the mean of the distances of each somatotype from the mean somatotype as plotted in three dimensions in component units [*Duquet and Hebbelinck*, 1977]. Thus, the SDI and SAM give the magnitude of the average scatter of somatotypes about their mean. For comparisons between separate variables t or F ratios have been used. For comparisons between some mean somatotypes taken as whole ratings, special analyses have been calculated using somatotype attitudinal distances (SAD) [*Carter*, 1980b; *Duquet and Hebbelinck*, 1977]. Using these methods, differences between dispersions about mean somatotypes, or between mean somatotypes, can be tested statistically. The somatotype categories referred to in this paper are those defined in *Carter* [1980b].

The samples for this paper are drawn from club, regional, national, and Olympic competitors. Information on the samples from the 1968 Olympic Games in Mexico City (MEXOG) is given in *de Garay* et al. [1974]. The sports represented in the MEXOG study are canoeing, diving, gymnastics, swimming, and track and field, with a total of 140 subjects. Another larger group of female athletes (n = 148) were studied at the 1976 Olympic Games in Montreal as part of the Montreal Olympic Games Anthropological Project (MOGAP). The larger samples were from canoeing, gymnastics, rowing, swimming, and

Table 1. Age, size, and somatotype of female Olympic athletes and reference samples

Sample	n	Statistic	Age years	Height cm	Weight kg	$\dfrac{\text{Height}}{\text{weight}^{1/3}}$	Endomorphy	Mesomorphy	Ectomorphy	SDI[a]	SAM[b]
1968 Mexico City Olympics (5 sports)	140	x̄	19.5	163.8	57.1	43.13	2.8	4.0	3.0	3.2	1.5
		s	4.23	7.78	9.26	1.38	1.14	0.87	0.96	2.19	0.93
1976 Montreal Olympics (5 sports)	90	x̄	19.0	166.9	56.9	43.51	2.6	3.7	3.3	3.0	1.3
		s	4.05	6.78	7.65	1.27	0.80	0.87	0.93	1.80	0.73
1976 Montreal Olympics (all sports)	148	x̄	20.9	169.6	60.8	43.24	2.8	3.8	3.1	3.0	1.3
		s	4.28	7.07	8.56	1.24	0.85	0.89	0.90	1.82	0.75
1968, Urban Mexicans	86	x̄	19.1	158.2	53.9	42.09	5.1	3.9	2.3	4.6	2.0
		s	3.50	6.40	7.60	1.92	1.64	0.99	1.19	2.31	0.99
1978, Canadian University Students	94	x̄	20.6	165.7	57.5	43.02	4.0	3.5	2.9	3.7	1.7
		s	2.60	6.10	6.37	1.37	1.25	0.95	0.98	1.93	0.83

[a] SDI = Somatotype dispersion index. [b] SAM = Somatotype attitudinal mean.

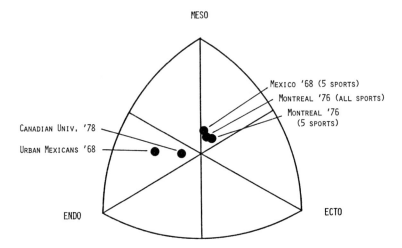

Fig. 1. Mean somatoplots of female Olympic athletes and reference samples.

track and field, with a few subjects each from basketball, diving, fencing, handball, and volleyball. The characteristics of the samples are given in each of the sections which follow. Data are presented for 16 sports, with a total of 87 samples (n = 1,770). They are drawn from studies covering the period from 1967 to 1980.

Athletes versus Non-Athletes

Do the somatotypes of Olympic athletes differ from reference samples of non-athletes? Attempting to answer this question poses some difficulties. Because the Olympic samples are made up of different sports, and the athletes are from different countries and ethnic backgrounds, and whereas the reference sample is usually from one country and of limited ethnic diversity, comparisons can only be made with these limitations in mind.

Comparisons were made between MEXOG athletes and 86 Urban Mexicans, and between the MOGAP sample and 94 Canadian University students (table I, fig. 1). The MEXOG athletes are significantly taller, heavier, less endomorphic, more ectomorphic, and had a smaller SAM than the Urban Mexicans. They are similar on age and mesomorphy. 40 of the Urban Mexicans were Caucasian and the remainder Mestizo. *Carter* et al. [1979] compared the 40 Caucasians with the 83 Caucasian athletes and showed that the athletes are taller and heavier, less endomorphic and more mesomorphic, but did not differ on ectomorphy, or on dispersions about their means (SAMs). The MOGAP athletes are taller, heavier, less endo-morphic, more mesomorphic, and have a smaller SAM than the Canadian University students [*Carter* et al., 1979]. There was better control of ethnic background in a study of CSSR university students and top female athletes in modern gymnastics, field handball, and track sprinting [*Stepnicka*, 1972]. His data show that the athletes were less endomorphic and more meso-morphic than the students. However, in contrast to the two Olympic com-parisons above, the CSSR samples did not differ on height or weight.

From these studies it is apparent that athletes as a group are less endo-morphic and more mesomorphic than non-athletes; however, these differ-ences are likely to depend upon the sports groups in the athletic sample as well as the ethnic composition of the athletes and non-athletes. Where single sports groups have been compared to suitable reference groups [*Carter* et al., 1979; *Day* et al., 1977; *Falls and Humphrey*, 1978; *Lebedeff*, 1980; *Step-nicka*, 1972, 1976a], or where they can be compared to reference samples from other studies, such as those reported in *Carter* [1980a], the somato-types of athletes are found to be different from non-athletes. The magnitude and direction of the differences on each component depend on the sport being compared.

Somatotypes of Athletes by Sport

Basketball

Studies on basketball players include samples of high school players from Austin, Texas [*Shoup*, 1978], teams from the University of Maryland [*Vaccaro* et al., 1979], and San Diego State University [*Robinson and Carter*, unpublished data], players from five teams in the 1974 Canadian Inter-collegiate Championships [*Alexander*, 1976], high level players in the USSR [*Carter*, 1970], and the Venezuelan national team [*Perez*, 1980]. The de-scriptive statistics are shown in table II and mean somatoplots on figure 2.

The mean somatoplots are near or to the left of the center of the somato-chart close to the ectomorphic axis. Four means have more mesomorphy than endomorphy, as have many subjects in these studies, while other sub-jects are meso-endomorphs, endo-mesomorphs, or endo-ectomorphs. Two means are in the central somatotype category. *Alexander* [1976] compared the best 10 players with the remaining players and found that the best players were heavier and showed a more restricted somatoplot distribution, which seemed largely due to decreased variability on endomorphy. The

Table II. Age, size and somatotype of female basketball players

Sample, reference	n	Stat-istic	Age years	Height cm	Weight kg	Height / weight $^{1/3}$	Endo-morphy	Meso-morphy	Ecto-morphy
Venezuela	19	x̄	18.4	168.2	59.0	43.15	3.2	3.8	3.1
[*Perez*, 1980]		s	3.04	6.92	6.49	1.47	0.83	1.01	1.06
Canada	53	x̄	20.0	170.6	63.9	42.71	4.0	3.5	2.7
[*Alexander*, 1976]		s	1.63	5.92	5.47	1.45	0.74	0.93	1.04
Maryland	15	x̄	19.4	173.0	68.3	42.32	4.3	3.9	2.4
[*Vaccaro* et al., 1977]		s	1.07	9.09	7.79	–	1.24	0.47	0.90
San Diego S.U. 1978	9	x̄	21.2	173.1	66.3	42.82	3.3	3.5	2.8
[*Robinson and Carter*, unpubl.]		s	1.30	8.06	7.61	1.06	0.89	0.85	0.77
USSR	10	x̄	–	173.0	71.4	41.70a	4.3	4.5	3.0
[*Carter*, 1970]		s	–	2.03	8.65	–	0.60	0.40	0.69
Austin	18	x̄	16.3	165.2	57.2	42.88a	3.9	4.0	2.5
[*Shoup*, 1978]		s	1.1	6.7	4.9	–	0.9	0.9	1.8

a Calculated from mean values.

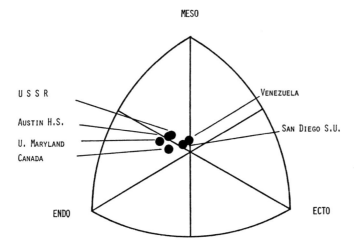

Fig. 2. Mean somatoplots of female basketball players.

mean somatotypes were similar (3.8–3.8–2.5 versus 4.1–3.4–2.8). There were no differences on size or somatotype components among the five teams.

Shoup [1978] plotted the means of his high school sample and a set of unpublished means provided by *Malina* for University of Texas players (n = 10, age = 20.0 years). The university sample had a mean somatoplot close to the 4–4–3 somatoplot and both samples were on the ectomorphic axis, but the high school players were approximately a half-unit less ectomorphic than the university players. The mean for the University of Texas players is close to those of other university means.

Chovanova and Zapletalova [1979] somatotyped the best young Czechoslovak teams at their National Championships in 1977–78. The age groups studied were: 13–14 years (n = 27); 15–16 years (n = 37); and 17–18 years (n = 32). They were also studied by playing position: guards (n = 45); forwards (n = 27); and centers (n = 24). Body size increased with age and from guards, through forwards to centers. The guards were the most mesomorphic and the centers the most ectomorphic. Most of the 13- to 14-year-olds were endomesomorphs, most of the 15- to 16-year-olds were central somatotypes, and for the 17- to 18-year-olds, the guards and forwards were in the central category and the centers were endo-ectomorphs. These findings suggest a shift from endo-mesomorphs to central somatotypes with increasing age. No such shift is apparent in the samples from different countries shown in table II. The two youngest samples (from Austin and Venezuela) are also the shortest and lightest.

Table III. Somatotypes of female gymnasts

Sample, reference	n	Statistic	Age years	Height cm	Weight kg	Height/weight$^{1/3}$	Endomorphy	Mesomorphy	Ectomorphy
Mexico City, 1968 [de Garay et al., 1974]	21	x̄	17.8	156.9	49.8	42.91	2.7	4.2	2.8
		s	3.7	5.1	4.5	0.73	0.70	0.46	0.53
Montreal, 1976	15	x̄	17.0	161.5	50.9	43.67	2.1	4.0	3.4
		s	2.0	5.7	6.0	1.00	0.43	0.61	0.74
Venezuela [Perez, 1980]	10	x̄	13.0	151.7	43.4	43.01	2.2	4.4	3.0
		s	1.56	6.86	7.24	1.17	0.66	0.61	0.92
Gama Filho [Araujo and Moutinho, 1978]	9	x̄	12.2	145.8	35.1	44.47[a]	1.8	3.3	4.1
		s	1.86	8.26	5.36	–	0.35	0.72	0.70
Springfield [Sinning, 1978]	44	x̄	19.4	160.6	53.7	42.57[a]	2.7[a]	3.6[a]	2.6[a]
		s	1.07	4.36	5.86	–	–	–	–
AIAW (NP) [Falls and Humphrey, 1978]	57	x̄	19.3	162.1	55.2	42.57	3.1	4.0	2.6
		s	0.98	5.08	4.73	–	0.63	0.78	0.74
AIAW (P) [Falls and Humphrey, 1978]	14	x̄	19.4	161.5	55.1	42.44	2.6	4.4	2.6
		s	1.50	4.65	5.77	–	0.81	0.8	0.68
USSR [Carter, 1970]	5	x̄	–	157.0	53.9	41.56[a]	3.8	5.2	1.6
		s	–	5.24	5.8	–	0.42	0.78	0.63
San Diego (club) [Strong, 1980]	20	x̄	14.8	156.0	46.8	43.31	2.5	3.5	3.4
		s	1.1	8.1	6.7	1.29	0.5	0.7	1.0
California, NQ [Strong, 1980]	13	x̄	13.9	150.8	42.2	43.41	1.7	4.2	3.1
		s	0.82	8.35	6.40	1.08	0.39	0.63	0.71
California, SQ [Strong, 1980]	28	x̄	13.6	153.8	44.3	43.53	2.0	3.9	3.3
		s	0.91	6.16	4.8	1.02	0.54	0.54	0.77
Munich, 1972 [Novak et al., 1977]	5	x̄	19.0	163.5	52.5	43.66[a]	2.6[a]	3.8[a]	3.4[a]
		s	3.5	2.3	1.2	–	–	–	–
French-Canada [Salmela, 1979]	7	x̄	13.9	142.6	35.6	43.35[a]	1.6[a]	4.4[a]	3.1[a]
		s	1.78	10.1	7.8	–	–	–	–
French-Canada [Salmela, 1979]	7	x̄	15.3	147.8	39.7	43.33[a]	1.5[a]	4.3[a]	3.1[a]
		s	1.78	9.3	7.4	–	–	–	–
Brno [Stepnicka, 1976 a, b]	17	x̄	12.5	147.8	37.0	44.35[a]	1.4	3.8	3.9
		s	–	5.7	5.10	–	0.56	0.56	0.74

[a] Calculated from mean values.

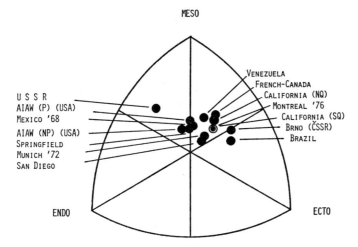

Fig. 3. Mean somatoplots of female gymnasts.

Gymnastics

The samples range from club to Olympic levels. The Olympic samples include the MEXOG gymnasts [*de Garay* et al., 1974], an Olympic team at Munich from one country [*Novak* et al., 1977], and the MOGAP gymnasts. National teams are represented by Venezuelans [*Perez*, 1980], and French-Canadians [*Salmela*, 1979], and other samples from studies by *Araujo and Moutinho* [1978] on young Brazilian club gymnasts, *Carter* [1970] on USSR club gymnasts, *Falls and Humphrey* [1978] on competitors in the 1974 AIAW Regional Championships in Springfield, Miss., *Sinning* [1978] on Springfield College gymnasts over a 5-year period, *Strong* [1980] on class I gymnasts at the club, state and national qualifying levels in California, and *Stepnicka* [1976a, b] on 12-year-old gymnasts from Brno, CSSR (table III, fig. 3).

Figure 3 shows that the mean somatoplots are primarily in the meso-morphic sector of the somatochart, but they range from endo-mesomorphy through balanced mesomorphy to the ectomorph-mesomorph category. Several factors may contribute to this variation. There is a wide range of age and physical maturity among the samples, the style and demands of Olympic gymnastics have changed in the past decade, and the samples have different ethnic backgrounds. For the Olympic gymnasts, the means for the 1972 and 1976 samples are similar, but the 1968 sample is more endo-mesomorphic with a mean close to the 3–4–3 somatotype. The 1976 distribution contains only 1 somatotype to the left of the mesomorphic axis, while there are 7 in the 1968 sample. The 1976 sample has an ellipsoid distribution while that of the 1968 sample is circular. The differences between the distributions suggest that the best gymnasts of recent Olympics may be more ectomorphic and less endomorphic than before. Within the 1968 sample, the Whites had a mean somatotype of 2.5–4.1–3.0, and the Mestizos 3.1–4.4–2.6 [*de Garay* et al., 1974]. Thus, Whites were ecto-mesomorphic and the Mestizos endo-mesomorphic. The 5 best gymnasts (CSSR team, bronze medal) were White, and were to the right of the mesomorphic axis.

7 of the 15 gymnasts at Montreal were from Italy and the remainder from Belgium, West Germany and the Netherlands. The somatotype means were: Italy = 2.1–3.8–3.2; others = 2.1–4.1–3.6. There were no differences between the mean somatotypes ($F = 0.80$, n.s.) or the dispersion means ($F = 0.08$, n.s.). Thus the Italian team had similar somatotypes to the northern Europeans.

The USSR sample probably represents gymnasts of the early 1960s, while the USA university samples are close to the somatotype mean of the MEXOG sample. *Strong's* [1980] study showed that as the level of competition increased from club to state and national qualifying levels the somatotype means became more ecto-mesomorphic. The best gymnasts had somatotypes similar to those of the MOGAP sample. The Brno and the Rio de Janiero samples are the youngest and most ectomorphic of all samples and are similar to each other. If there is a trend it seems to be that the most recent samples, and samples of the youngest and best are concentrated in the ecto-mesomorphic category, with others in the balanced mesomorphy and ectomorph-mesomorph categories. Examination of the somatocharts of the samples shows that most of the distributions are elliptical with little variation on endomorphy.

Ross et al. [1978] showed that for persons of short stature, the criterion photoscopic rating of endomorphy was underestimated by about a half-unit when derived from the skinfolds without a correction based upon stature. Because gymnasts are quite short the endomorphic ratings in table III are probably underestimated. If the correction, anthropometric endomorphy × (170.18 cm/stature in cm), is applied to the values in table III, the endomorphy component means are increased from 0.1 to 0.3 units.

Skating

Ross et al. [1977a], and *Faulkner* [1976], studied the somatotypes of the best Canadian figure skaters in different performance categories: Senior and Junior Ladies (n = 18); Novice Ladies (n = 9); outstanding skaters over

Table IV. Age, size and somatotype of female skaters and skiers

Sample, reference	n	Statistic	Age years	Height cm	Weight kg	Height / weight$^{1/3}$	Endo- morphy	Meso- morphy	Ecto- morphy
Skaters									
Canada (S-JL) [Ross et al., 1977a]	18	x̄	15.7	156.8	48.6	42.97[a]	2.6	3.8	3.0
		s	1.58	5.2	6.1	–	0.7	0.6	0.9
Canada (NL) [Ross et al., 1977a]	9	x̄	13.2	153.5	42.1	44.12[a]	2.1	3.7	3.9
		s	1.38	8.9	5.7	–	0.4	0.7	0.7
Canada (12+) [Faulkner, 1976]	21	x̄	14.0	154.1	45.5	43.17[a]	2.5	4.1	3.2
		s	1.7	8.5	8.2	–	0.7	0.5	0.9
Canada (12−) [Faulkner, 1976]	12	x̄	10.7	136.7	31.2	43.42[a]	2.5	4.2	3.3
		s	1.1	9.4	5.6	–	0.7	0.6	1.0
Skiers									
USA Nordic [Sinning et al., 1977]	5	x̄	23.5	164.5	56.9	42.77[a]	3.5	4.3	2.3
		s	4.66	3.25	1.09	–	0.71	0.45	0.84
Rossland, Downhill [Ross and Day, 1972]	15	x̄	10.7	139.7	32.7	43.69[a]	2.0	4.0	3.6
		s	2.17	13.9	8.75	–	0.53	0.85	1.13
CSSR Downhill [Stepnicka and Broda, 1977]	11	x̄	13.0	156.4	48.2	42.98[a]	2.5	4.3	3.0
		s	–	6.77	7.62	–	0.86	0.23	0.72

[a] Calculated from mean values.

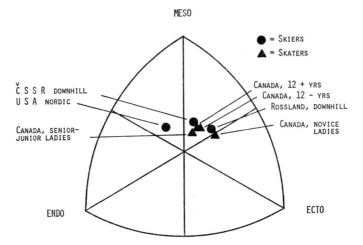

MESO

● = SKIERS
▲ = SKATERS

v̌
C S S R DOWNHILL
U S A NORDIC

CANADA, 12 + YRS
CANADA, 12 - YRS
ROSSLAND, DOWNHILL

CANADA, NOVICE
LADIES

CANADA, SENIOR-
JUNIOR LADIES

ENDO   ECTO

Fig. 4. Mean somatoplots of female skaters and skiers.

12 years of age (n = 21); and outstanding skaters under 12 years of age (n = 12) (table IV, fig. 4). The mean ages ranged from 10.7 to 15.7 years and the body size increased from the youngest to the oldest group as would be expected. The mean somatoplots of the under and over 12-year-olds are almost identical (approximately 2.5–4–3), while the Novice Ladies are close to the 2–4–4 and the Senior-Junior Ladies are similar to the under and over 12-year-olds. Also reported was the somatotype of world champion Karen Magnussen (3.5–4.5–2.5). Her somatotype and those of the three top-rated skaters in the study were slightly to the left of the mean somatoplot of the groups. The authors suggest that with increasing age movement of the somatotype in the direction of increased endomorphy may reflect a normal female growth phenomenon accompanying physical maturation. Young skaters appear to have similar somatotypes to young gymnasts.

Skiing

Two groups of young downhill skiers have been studied. *Ross and Day* [1972] somatotyped 15 Nancy Greene Ski League competitive skiers 6–14 years of age at Rossland, B.C. *Stepnicka and Broda* [1977] somatotyped the best CSSR downhill skiers 12–14 years of age (table IV, fig. 4). The CSSR skiers were older and larger, more endomorphic and mesomorphic, and less ectomorphic than the Rossland skiers. Some of these differences are probably due to age. The majority of both samples were dominant in mesomorphy, and their distributions are similar to those of young gymnasts.

Table V. Age, size, and somatotype of female swimmers

Sample, reference	n	Statistic	Age years	Height cm	Weight kg	Height/weight$^{1/3}$	Endo-morphy	Meso-morphy	Ecto-morphy
Mexico City, 1968 [Hebbelinck et al., 1975]	27	x̄	16.3	164.4	56.9	43.08	3.1	4.0	3.0
		s	2.9	7.1	9.1	1.22	0.9	0.7	0.9
Montreal, 1976	32	x̄	16.6	166.9	57.8	43.24	3.2	3.8	3.0
		s	2.62	5.7	6.83	1.24	0.78	0.71	0.89
Munich, 1972 [Novak et al., 1976]	7	x̄	17.7	167.0	60.1	42.63[a]	3.2[a]	4.6[a]	2.6[a]
		s	2.3	8.9	7.7	–	–	–	–
Venezuela [Perez, 1980]	14	x̄	14.8	163.7	55.2	42.65	3.2	4.1	2.8
		s	1.18	4.54	4.37	1.35	1.08	0.83	0.95
Brazil [Rocha et al., 1977]	15	x̄	16.3	166.0	59.6	42.52	3.3	3.5	2.9
		s	1.67	4.48	4.61	1.06	0.73	0.47	0.88
Manchester [Bagnall et al., 1977]	12	x̄	15.3	–	54.3	–	2.1	3.8	3.5
		s	–	–	–	–	0.5	0.9	0.8
Austin [Shoup, 1978]	41	x̄	17.1	168.2	56.0	44.00	2.9	3.7	3.6
		s	2.44	6.3	4.7	1.11	0.84	0.82	0.81
Caracas [Perez, 1977]	12	x̄	13.8	158.2	46.5	43.99[a]	2.3	3.8	3.4
		s	–	–	–	–	1.10	1.04	1.63
Chula Vista AAU, 1976 [Krogh et al., unpubl.]	15	x̄	14.2	161.3	52.2	43.1	2.4	3.4	2.8
		s	0.96	5.33	2.11	0.93	0.50	0.73	0.88
San Diego S.U., 1976 [Krogh et al., unpubl.]	15	x̄	19.5	169.0	65.9	41.99	3.9	3.8	2.2
		s	1.25	6.98	9.83	1.82	1.14	1.13	1.29
San Diego S.U., 1978 [Atchley et al., unpubl.]	15	x̄	19.5	169.6	61.8	42.85	3.9	4.1	2.80
		s	1.06	6.81	6.84	1.69	0.90	1.02	1.24

[a] Calculated from mean values.

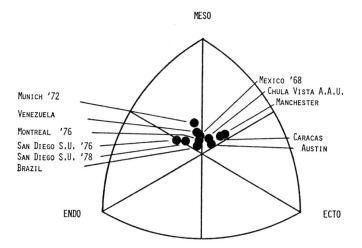

Fig. 5. Mean somatoplots of female swimmers.

The only adult sample reported is the USA Nordic ski team of 1976 [*Sinning* et al., 1977]. Their mean somatotype is endo-mesomorphic, approximately 3.5–4.5–2.5, and all 5 somatotypes are in the north-eastern sector of the somatochart.

Swimming

The club samples are from Austin, Tex. [*Meleski* et al., 1980], Caracas, Venezuela [*Perez*, 1977], Chula Vista, USA [*Krogh and Kreshka*, unpublished data], and Manchester, England [*Bagnall and Kellett*, 1977]; National teams are represented by Brazilians [*Rocha* et al., 1977], Venezuelans [*Perez*, 1980], and Olympic samples by MEXOG [*de Garay* et al., 1974; *Hebbelinck* et al., 1975], Munich [*Novak* et al., 1977], and MOGAP. Two teams (1976 and 1978) from San Diego State University are also represented (table V, fig. 5) [*Krogh, Keshka, and Atchley*, unpublished data].

The mean ages range from 13.8 to 17.7 years, and some samples have wide ranges (e.g. the Austin sample ranges from 11 to 20 years). The mean somatoplots cluster in or near the 3–4–3 somatotype, and in a broad area between the 4–4–2 and the 2–4–4 somatoplots. The club teams seem to be the least endomorphic and the university teams (who are also the oldest) are the most endomorphic. The means for the three Olympic samples are similar and near the 3.5–4–3 somatotype. The majority of physiques in these

Table VI. Age, size and somatotype of female tennis players

Sample, reference	n	Statistic	Age years	Height cm	Weight kg	Height / weight$^{1/3}$	Endo- morphy	Meso- morphy	Ecto- morphy
USA College [Lebedeff, 1980]	14	x̄	20.4	166.4	57.9	43.1	4.6	3.9	3.0
		s	0.84	7.17	7.69	0.77	1.00	1.02	0.57
College B [Lebedeff, 1980]	14	x̄	19.9	169.7	62.0	43.1	5.7	2.6	3.1
		s	1.34	6.07	9.62	2.24	1.35	1.75	1.31
USA Juniors [Lebedeff, 1980]	21	x̄	16.7	166.3	59.0	42.8	4.0	4.0	2.7
		s	1.42	7.30	7.53	1.31	0.94	0.89	0.91
Professionals [Copley, 1980]	19	x̄	24.1	167.3	60.7	42.57[a]	3.1	3.9	2.6
		s	4.49	4.66	6.02	–	1.26	1.00	0.87
Amateurs [Copley, 1980]	11	x̄	24.9	167.9	55.4	44.04[a]	2.6	3.2	3.6
		s	11.51	5.04	4.31	–	0.80	0.96	0.80

[a] Calculated from mean values.

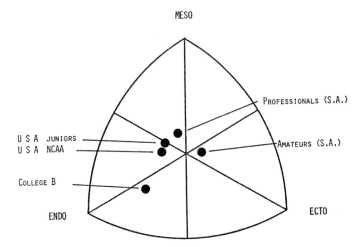

Fig. 6. Mean somatoplots of female tennis players.

samples are central, or endo-mesomorphic. For the MEXOG sample the freestyle swimmers were more ectomorphic than the breaststroke, backstroke, or medley swimmers [*de Garay* et al., 1974; *Hebbelinck* et al., 1975]. The distributions for both the MEXOG and MOGAP samples are almost circular with considerable overlapping, when the MOGAP swimmers are compared by stroke (freestyle, $n = 11$; breaststroke, $n = 5$; backstroke, $n = 7$, and butterfly, $n = 9$), there are no differences among somatotype means ($F = 0.70$, n.s.), among mean dispersions ($F = 0.82$, n.s.), or on weight ($F = 2.42$, n.s.). However, butterfly swimmers are older than freestyle and backstroke swimmers ($F = 5.69$, sign.), and breaststrokers are taller than butterfly swimmers ($F = 3.80$, sign.).

The Francisco de Miranda Club team [*Perez*, 1977] showed wide variation in somatotypes with one third of the somatoplots well to the left of the mesomorphic axis, but the Manchester Club have less variability and are all to the right of the mesomorphy axis. When the Chula Vista AAU swimmers were compared to the 1976 San Diego State University swimmers, the club swimmers were younger, shorter, lighter, less endomorphic and more ectomorphic [*Krogh and Keshka*, unpublished data]. *Rocha* et al. [1977] studied other swimmers at the 'international level' ($n = 44$) and found them to be similar in age, size, and somatotype among strokes and events to the 1975 Brazilian selection.

Tennis

Copley [1980] and *Lebedeff* [1980] studied tennis players at different levels of competition (table VI, fig. 6). *Copley* [1980] somatotyped 19 professional and 11 amateur players competing in the 1977 South African Open Tennis Championships. The professionals were heavier, more mesomorphic and less ectomorphic than the amateurs. *Lebedeff* [1980] somatotyped competitors in the 1976 USTA Women's National Collegiate Championships, local university players (College B), and Juniors (under 18 years of age) competing in the National City Team Championships in 1977. She found that the Junior and National Collegiate players were similar in size and somatotype and both were less endomorphic and more mesomorphic than the College B players. The Junior and National Collegiate players were similar in size and somatotype to *Copley's* professionals. The somatoplots of all samples about their means were roughly circular.

Track and Field

Descriptive statistics are shown in table VII and somatoplots in figures 7–9. The samples are arranged by event groupings, except that data for all competitors from MEXOG and MOGAP are combined at the beginning of the table. *Guimaraes and De Rose* [1978, 1980] reported the results of their study on the size and somatotype of track and field athletes participating in the National Student Games in Porto Alegre, 1976, and Brasilia, 1977. The participants were less than 18 years of age. The results from the two studies are combined (n = 203) in table VII and on the somatocharts. Other samples include San Diego County athletes [*Westlake*, 1967], Austin high schooll runners [*Shoup*, 1978], middle distance runners competing in Munich [*Novak* et al., 1977], Venezuelan sprinters and hurdlers [*Perez*, 1980], CSSR sprinters [*Stepnicka*, 1972], and European and Belgian middle and long-distance runners [*Day* et al., 1977].

Sprinters and Hurdlers (table VII, fig. 7). The mean somatoplots are to the northeast of the ectomorphic axis on the somatochart around the central category. There appears to be a slight shift in the mean somatoplot from 1968 to 1976 in the Olympic samples. The 1976 sample is less endomorphic and mesomorphic and more ectomorphic than the 1968 sample. Both the MEXOG and CSSR samples had a large number of subjects in the endomesomorphy category. *Hirata* [1979] plotted the somatotypes of nine sprinters from Chukyo University and their mean was approximately 4–5–1, much more endo-mesomorphic than those reported in this review.

Table VII. Age, size, and somatotype of female track and field athletes

Sample, reference	n	Statistic	Age years	Height cm	Weight kg	Height / weight^(1/3)	Endo- morphy	Meso- morphy	Ecto- morphy
Mexico City, 1968 [de Garay et al., 1974]	82	X̄	20.8	168.0	59.2	43.28	2.8	3.8	3.1
		s	3.6	7.5	9.7	1.55	1.40	0.96	1.05
Montreal, 1976	34	X̄	21.8	168.5	57.2	43.84	2.3	3.4	3.5
		s	3.73	7.09	7.66	1.44	0.71	1.02	1.04
Sprinters and Hurdlers									
Mexico City, 1968 [de Garay et al., 1974]	28	X̄	20.7	165.0	56.8	43.01	2.7	3.9	2.9
		s	3.4	6.3	6.6	1.09	0.93	0.66	0.80
Montreal, 1976	7	X̄	22.8	165.9	55.1	46.63	2.2	3.4	3.4
		s	3.39	6.22	4.43	1.18	0.49	0.79	0.90
Venezuela [Perez, 1980]	7	X̄	20.7	164.8	51.7	44.18	2.3	2.9	3.8
		s	4.23	4.89	4.20	1.09	0.39	0.67	0.69
Brazil, 1976–77 [Guimaraes et al., 1978, 1980]	62	X̄	16.5	160.6	50.1	43.56	2.9	3.4	3.4
		s	1.41	4.35	4.14	–	0.88	0.80	0.78
CSSR [Stepnicka, 1972]	49	X̄	–	166.7	60.1	42.74[a]	3.4	4.3	2.7
		s	–	4.58	6.19	–	0.81	0.40	0.98
San Diego County [Westlake, 1967]	24	X̄	16.7	168.4	54.2	44.63	3.0	3.3	4.0
		s	1.89	5.74	4.18	1.72	0.74	1.04	1.43
400 m									
Mexico City, 1968	11	X̄	19.5	165.4	53.4	43.97	2.0	3.4	3.6
		s	2.62	6.61	4.33	1.02	0.63	0.64	0.77

Table VII. (continued)

Sample, reference	n	Statistic	Age years	Height cm	Weight kg	Height weight$^{1/3}$	Endo-morphy	Meso-morphy	Ecto-morphy
Brazil, HJ. [Guimaraes et al., 1978, 1980]	11	x̄	17.1	174.7	56.0	45.66[a]	2.8	2.0	4.9
		s	1.19	4.54	5.37	–	0.66	0.66	0.75
Brazil, LJ. [Guimaraes et al., 1978, 1980]	16	x̄	16.0	164.5	51.9	44.10[a]	3.0	3.2	3.6
		s	1.18	4.22	4.36	–	0.86	0.80	1.73
San Diego, H+LJ. [Westlake, 1967]	12	x̄	17.3	168.2	52.0	45.16	2.9	2.9	4.5
		s	1.72	6.53	5.40	1.36	0.67	0.62	1.02
Mexico City, S+D [de Garay et al., 1974]	9	x̄	19.9	170.9	73.5	40.93	5.3	5.2	1.7
		s	4.3	8.3	12.6	2.08	1.97	1.39	1.14
Brazil, S+D. [Guimaraes et al., 1978]	19	x̄	17.3	166.5	67.1	40.97[a]	5.0	4.5	1.5
		s	1.00	5.60	7.55	–	0.70	1.05	1.10
San Diego, S, D, J. [Westlake, 1967]	13	x̄	18.2	168.3	69.0	41.39	5.2	4.7	2.2
		s	2.11	7.47	15.22	2.44	1.78	1.42	1.45
Mexico City, J. [de Garay et al., 1974]	4	x̄	20.2	180.1	73.1	43.34	3.6	3.7	3.1
		s	3.4	5.5	16.8	2.35	1.70	1.26	1.6
Brazil, J. [Guimaraes et al., 1978]	8	x̄	17.2	169.7	64.7	42.27[a]	4.4	3.6	2.5
		s	1.1	4.9	8.9	–	1.1	1.5	0.7
Mexico City, P. [de Garay et al., 1974]	11	x̄	22.5	169.5	60.0	43.37	2.4	3.6	3.1
		s	4.4	7.4	7.4	0.93	0.79	0.73	0.66
Brazil, P. [Guimaraes et al., 1978, 1980]	12	x̄	17.8	169.5	57.1	44.02[a]	3.0	3.0	3.7
		s	0.82	7.48	7.38	–	0.81	1.26	1.00

[a] Calculated from mean values.

[b] The capital letters refer to events: H = high jump; L = long jump; S = shot put; D = discus throw; J = javelin throw; P = pentathlon.

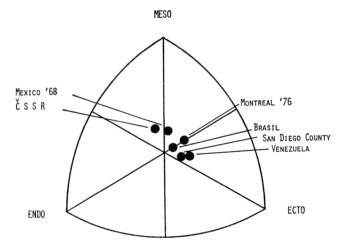

Fig. 7. Mean somatoplots of female sprinters and hurdlers.

400 Meters (table VII, fig. 8). The MEXOG and MOGAP runners are almost identical in somatotype (approximately 2–3.5–3.5) but the young Brazilians are more central at 3–3–3.5).

800 through 3,000 Meters (table VII, fig. 8). The best samples have remarkably similar somatotypes. The MEXOG, MOGAP, Munich, European and Belgian runners at these distances have somatoplots in a small triangular area bounded by the somatotypes 3–4–4, 2–4–4, and 2–3–4. The Brazilians (800 and 1,500 m), San Diego County runners (400–1,650 m), and the Austin runners (sprinters through long-distance) are all more endomorphic than the other samples. *Day* et al. [1977] reported little difference between the 800- and the 1,500- to 3,000-m subgroups of their European and Belgian samples. The mean somatoplots of all groups were close together with the Europeans slightly less endomorphic than the Belgians.

Field Events (table VII, fig. 9). Field events included throwing, jumping and the pentathlon. Mean somatoplots are along or near the ectomorphic axis from the northwest end (shot and discus throwers) to the southeast (high jumpers). The javelin throwers, pentathlonists, and long jumpers lie in an intermediate position along the axis. The three samples of long jumpers are near the 2.5–3.5–3.5 somatoplot, which is also close to that of the sprinters. The mean somatoplots for the pentathlon are close to the long

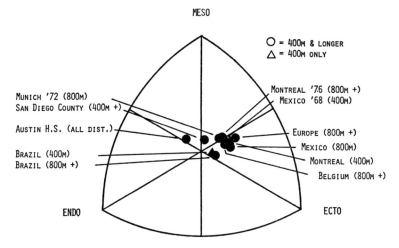

Fig. 8. Mean somatoplots of female middle- and long-distance runners.

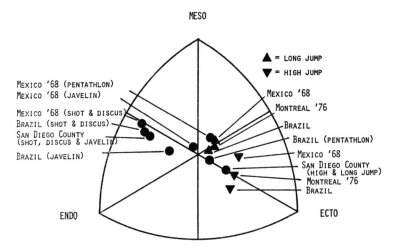

Fig. 9. Mean somatoplots of female field event competitors.

jump means, but the young Brazilians are less mesomorphic than the MEXOG athletes.

Within the Brazilian group there is little differentiation among the means for the runners, long jumpers, and pentathlonists, but the high jumpers, shot putters and discus throwers, and javelin throwers have quite

Table VIII. Age, size and somatotype of female athletes from various sports

Samples, reference	n	Statistic	Age years	Height cm	Weight kg	$\dfrac{\text{Height}}{\text{weight}^{1/3}}$	Endo-morphy	Meso-morphy	Ecto-morphy
Canoeing [de Garay et al., 1974]	4	x̄	22.0	163.1	61.0	41.42	3.5	5.3	1.8
		s	2.7	3.9	2.8	0.53	0.94	0.56	0.43
Canoeing, Montreal, 1976	8	x̄	20.6	170.7	63.0	42.98	2.8	4.1	2.9
		s	5.14	6.86	8.03	0.78	0.26	0.78	0.58
Diving [de Garay et al., 1974]	7	x̄	21.1	160.4	52.3	42.94	2.9	4.0	2.9
		s	7.6	2.9	3.9	0.79	0.80	0.64	0.48
Golf, Professional [Carter, 1971]	26	x̄	27.8	167.6	62.4	42.48	4.1	4.0	2.7
		s	7.9	7.19	8.23	0.53	1.11	1.11	1.11
Golf, Amateur [Carter, 1971]	26	x̄	40.5	164.8	62.9	41.33	4.9	4.6	2.1
		s	8.66	4.90	6.46	0.60	1.0	1.3	1.1
Gymnastics (modern) [Stepnicka, 1972]	71	x̄	–	163.5	57.1	42.52	3.6	4.3	2.6
		s	–	4.23	4.38	–	0.89	0.52	0.78
Handball (field) [Stepnicka, 1972]	78	x̄	–	165.6	62.0	41.86	4.1	4.3	2.3
		s	–	4.92	6.00	–	1.01	0.48	0.94
Rowing, Montreal, 1976	51	x̄	23.8	174.3	67.4	42.88	3.1	3.9	2.8
		s	2.65	4.78	5.33	1.00	0.84	0.87	0.78
Surfboard riding [Lowdon, 1980]	14	x̄	21.6	165.7	59.3	42.49	3.9	4.1	2.6
		s	3.35	4.91	6.70	–	1.08	0.66	0.84
Synchronized swimming [Ross, unpubl. 1978]	136	x̄	16.8	163.8	53.2	43.70	3.3	3.6	3.4
		s	2.27	7.2	7.5	1.58	1.04	0.89	1.14
Volleyball (Venezuela) [Perez, 1980]	11	x̄	20.1	165.1	58.8	42.35	3.3	4.1	2.5
		s	2.94	3.60	3.74	1.39	0.56	0.97	0.96
Volleyball (Austin) [Shoup, 1978]	43	x̄	16.1	165.0	59.4	42.29	4.7	4.0	2.6
		s	1.1	8.5	9.8	–	1.3	1.0	1.4

Table VIII (continued)

Group	n								
Montreal, 1976	7	x̄	21.1	167.9	56.0	44.00	1.8	3.2	3.6
		s	2.86	7.09	7.20	1.12	0.39	0.95	0.73
Brazil, 1976–77	38	x̄	16.1	161.6	49.9	43.89[a]	2.9	3.2	3.6
		s	1.96	6.2	4.87	–	0.65	0.85	0.85
[*Guimaraes* et al., 1978, 1980]									
800 m and longer									
Brazil, 800+1,500 m	36	x̄	15.9	159.9	48.1	43.97[a]	3.0	3.1	3.7
		s	1.39	4.76	5.32	–	0.92	0.79	0.98
[*Guimaraes* et al., 1978, 1980]									
Mexico City, 1968	7	x̄	20.9	169.2	55.6	44.40	2.1	3.2	3.9
		s	3.2	4.36	3.91	0.95	0.89	0.70	0.80
Montreal, 1976	6	x̄	20.6	163.5	52.5	43.75	2.1	3.5	3.4
		s	3.63	6.27	6.90	0.72	0.59	0.71	0.59
800+1,500 m									
Europe, 800–3,000 m	33	x̄	24.14	164.86	52.27	44.09[a]	1.7	3.4	3.7
		s	4.17	4.73	3.86	–	0.52	0.71	0.81
[*Day* et al., 1977]									
Belgium, 800–3,000 m	33	x̄	19.09	163.77	51.58	44.00[a]	2.3	3.5	3.7
		s	3.19	5.25	4.95	–	0.50	0.63	0.81
[*Day* et al., 1977]									
Other groups									
Austin, Sprint and distance	25	x̄	16.8	162.2	54.3	42.83[a]	3.7	3.8	2.7
		s	1.1	6.9	7.1	–	1.2	0.7	1.0
[*Shoup*, 1978]									
San Diego, 400–1,650 m	12	x̄	16.9	162.3	52.1	43.41	3.1	3.8	3.3
		s	2.17	4.90	3.59	1.65	0.96	0.90	0.99
[*Westlake*, 1967]									
Munich, 400–1,500 m	8	x̄	24.2	167.6	57.0	43.55[a]	2.2[a]	3.4[a]	3.3[a]
		s	3.8	7.7	7.1	–	–	–	–
[*Novak* et al., 1977]									
Field events [b]									
Mexico City, H+LJ	12	x̄	21.5	169.4	56.4	44.27	2.2	3.3	3.7
		s	4.1	7.7	4.3	1.16	0.54	0.68	0.89
[*de Garay* et al., 1974]									
Montreal, H+LJ	10	x̄	21.6	173.6	58.0	44.86	2.4	2.7	4.3
		s	4.75	6.07	3.66	1.12	0.24	0.89	0.82

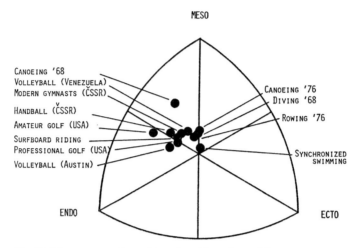

Fig. 10. Mean somatoplots of female athletes from different sports.

different means. In general, these samples of young Brazilians are more endomorphic and less mesomorphic than the Olympic samples.

de Garay et al. [1974] reported significant differences among event groups in track and field for all three somatotype components. The shot and discus throwers were more endomorphic, mesomorphic and less ecto-morphic than sprinters, middle-distance runners, jumpers, or pentathlonists. Also, javelin throwers were more endomorphic than middle-distance runners and jumpers, and the sprinters more mesomorphic and less ectomorphic than the middle-distance runners and jumpers. The sprinters were shorter than the shot and discus throwers and the javelin throwers, and the latter were taller than all other groups. The throwers were clearly heavier than the other event groups, and of these groups the middle-distance runners were lighter than the pentathlonists.

Other Sports

Descriptive statistics and the somatochart for these sports are shown in table VIII and figure 10.

Canoeing. MEXOG and MOGAP samples are available for Olympic canoeists. There is a large difference between the mean somatoplots for the 1968 and 1976 Olympics, but the numbers are small and there were some event differences between the Olympics. It is difficult to ascertain if this is a true shift or a sampling problem. 2 of the MEXOG sample were rated at six in mesomorphy, while the highest rating in the MOGAP sample was five for 2 subjects.

Diving. The mean for the MEXOG sample is almost 3–4–3 and most somatotypes are in the central or balanced mesomorphy categories.

Golf. Two samples of golfers, professional and amateur, were somato-typed by *McClure* [1967] using the M.4 method. Heath-Carter anthro-pometric ratings were calculated later and reported by *Carter* [1971]. The amateur golfers were older, more endomorphic and mesomorphic and less ectomorphic than the professionals. Both groups had large numbers of endomorph-mesomorphs.

Modern Gymnastics. Modern gymnastics is a different form from Olym-pic gymnastics, which was reviewed above. This sample is from the study of *Stepnicka* [1972] of CSSR athletes. The modern gymnasts are more endo-morphic than the best samples of Olympic gymnasts.

Handball. The field handball sample is also from *Stepnicka* [1972]. These players are close to the 4–4–2 somatotype, and are more endomorphic than some of the other samples such as divers, rowers, and synchronized swimmers. *Stepnicka* et al. [1979b] somatotyped eight Junior teams during the International Handball Tournament Druzba in CSSR in 1977. The players averaged 170.0 cm in height, 64.7 kg in weight, and had a mean somatotype of 3.3–4.1–2.5. The teams only differed slightly from each other but there were greater differences by playing position.

Rowing. The first large group of rowers who have been somatotyped were those in the MOGAP sample [*Carter* et al., 1979]. These rowers were similar with respect to geographic origin, style, and event, with an average somatotype of 3–4–3. There were some differences on endomorphy. The USA eight was less endomorphic than the Canadian eight, and the eights and fours were more endomorphic than the singles and pairs.

Surfboard Riding. *Lowdon* [1980] somatotyped the best surfboard riders at a world professional surfing circuit competition in Australia. The top three riders were more ectomorphic than the less successful competitors, and resembled those of Olympic freestyle swimmers. The author noted that the three Australians were more mesomorphic and endomorphic, and less ectomorphic than those from Hawaii or the USA. The means were 5.0–4.7–1.7, 3.5–4.0–2.8, and 3.7–3.9–3.0, respectively.

Synchronized Swimming. The sample was somatotyped by *Ross* et al. [personal communication], at the Canadian Synchronized Swimming Championships in 1978. Their mean is at the center of the somatochart and the distribution of somatotypes around their mean is extensive indicating a wide range on each of the components. They seem to be slightly less mesomorphic than some of the high-quality swimming groups (table V, fig. 5).

Volleyball. Two samples are presented, the Venezuelan team [*Perez*, 1980] and players from five high schools in Austin, Tex. [*Shoup*, 1978]. The means show that the Venezuelans are endo-mesomorphs, and the Austin players are meso-endomorphs, with the largest difference being on endomorphy. The Venezuelans were less variable on endomorphy than on the other two components. *Shoup* [1978] plotted the means of his high school sample along with unpublished means from *Malina* for University of Texas players (n = 15, age = 19.9 years) and candidates for the USA Olympic Team in 1976 (n = 18, age = 22.5 years). The University mean was near the 5–3–2 somatoplot and the Olympic mean was near the 4–4–3 somatoplot (and almost the same as the University of Texas basketball players). *Vivolo* et al. [1978] reported that the Japanese National Team were endomorph-mesomorphs, with endomorphy 0.3 units higher than mesomorphy.

Somatotype Differences between Sports

In the previous section we have seen that there are some differences within sports. These differences may be due to such variables as level of competition, age of competitors, positions or events within sports. Examination of figures 2–10 shows that some sports have quite different mean somatoplots, while others are similar to each other. Several studies have compared athletes from different sports. *de Garay* et al. [1974] tested the differences on somatotype components among gymnasts, divers, canoeists, swimmers, sprinters and hurdlers, and shot and discus throwers. They found that the throwers and canoeists were more mesomorphic and less ectomorphic than the other sports groups, and that the throwers were more endomorphic than the others. The gymnasts, divers, swimmers, and sprinters were close to the 3–4–3 somatotype. The thrower's mean was near 5.5–5–1, and the canoeist's mean near 3.5–5.5–2.

Comparisons among sports were made using the MOGAP athletes for canoeing, gymnastics, swimming, rowing, and track and field. There were no differences among the dispersion means, but there were differences among the somatotype means. These differences were attributed to endomorphy. The gymnasts and track-and-field athletes were lower on endomorphy than the canoeists, rowers, or swimmers [Carter, unpublished data].

In their studies of CSSR athletes, Stepnicka [1972] and Stepnicka et al. [1979a] showed that modern gymnasts and track sprinters were approximately a half-unit lower on endomorphy and higher on ectomorphy than field handball players. All three groups were similar on mesomorphy. The gymnasts were shorter and lighter than either handball players or sprinters who did not differ from each other. Perez [1980] made comparisons among the Venezuelan teams for basketball, gymnastics, swimming, track sprinting, and volleyball. Sprinters and gymnasts had different mean somatotypes from the other three sports. The sprinters were more meso-ectomorphic than the other groups, and the gymnasts were more ecto-mesomorphic than the other groups. There were no differences among sports with respect to dispersion means.

The highest values on endomorphy are to be found in shot and discus throwers, and some golfers, tennis players, swimmers, and rowers, while the lowest values are found in distance runners, gymnasts, and high jumpers. The highest values on mesomorphy are found in the shot and discus throwers, some canoeists and rowers, while the lowest values are found in high jumpers, some distance runners, tennis players, and synchronized swimmers. The highest values on ectomorphy are found in high jumpers, some basketball and volleyball players, and distance runners, while the lowest values are found in shot and discus throwers.

Sexual Dimorphism and Somatotype

Sexual dimorphism based on mean somatotype differences has been observed between male and female non-athlete and athlete groups [Carter, 1974, 1978a, 1980a; Heath, 1977; Ross et al., 1977b]. Comparisons between male and female athletes in the same sports from the 1968 and 1976 Olympics demonstrate similar patterns [Carter, 1978b]. In general, there is sexual dimorphism within event, with the lines connecting the means running in a northeast to southwest direction on the somatochart. This means that the females are more endomorphic and less mesomorphic than the males with little difference on ectomorphy. These differences are similar to those in the general population except that both the male and female athlete samples are less endomorphic and more mesomorphic than the non-athletes. In other studies where male and female sport comparisons are available similar patterns of sexual dimorphism are seen [*Araujo and Moutinho*, 1978; *Bagnall and Kellett*, 1977; *Chovanova and Zapletalova*, 1979; *Faulkner*, 1976; *Guimaraes and De Rose*, 1978, 1980; *Hebbelinck* et al., 1975; *Lowdon*, 1980; *Perez*, 1980; *Rocha* et al., 1977; *Ross and Day*, 1972; *Ross* et al., 1977b; *Sinning* et al., 1977; *Stepnicka*, 1972, 1976a, b].

Summary and Conclusions

Somatotype studies of female athletes of different ages, levels of competition, sports and events, and from different countries have been reviewed and new data have been analyzed. Data are presented for 16 sports, 87 sport or event samples, based on 1,770 athletes. Several limitations should be considered when interpreting the findings in this review and making comparisons between samples: (1) some samples have different ethnic composition; (2) some samples are small and may not be representative of the sport or event, while others are large and probably include a wide range of abilities; (3) ability levels between samples may not be comparable; and (4) somatotype is but one method of quantifying structure, and structure is but one aspect of successful performance.

On the basis of previous studies and analysis of new data, the following findings summarize present knowledge about the somatotypes of female athletes: (1) Top class female athletes in most sports are more mesomorphic and less endomorphic than non-athletes. (2) Somatotypes of female athletes from the 1968 and 1976 Olympics are similar in some sports but there are possible differences in track sprinting, canoeing, and gymnastics. (3) Quite different somatotypes appear necessary for success in some sports, whereas there are similar somatotype distributions in other sports. (4) Somatotype means for different sports and events have a wide range along or near the ectomorphic axis of the somatochart. (5) Means for a large number of sports and events are in the somatochart area bounded by somatotypes 4–4–3, 3–4–3, 2–4–4, and 3–3–3. (6) Successful young female athletes have somatotypes similar to, or approaching, those of older athletes in most sports.

(7) Somatotype patterns for athletes of different sports within a country appear similar to those of other countries but sometimes differ slightly in magnitude due to possible age, training level, or ethnic differences. (8) Female athletes are less mesomorphic and more endomorphic than males in most sports. (9) Sexual dimorphism between mean somatotypes for athletes in the same sport is similar in magnitude and direction to that of non-athletes.

As reviewed in this paper, there is sufficient evidence to confirm the findings from studies on male athletes that there is a relationship between successful performance and somatotype. To be successful, female athletes should have (or should try to acquire) the appropriate somatotype which is characteristic of those who are already successful.

Acknowledgements

The author thanks his colleagues in the Montreal Olympic Games Anthropological Project, as well as *Barbara Heath* and *Stephen Aubry* for their assistance. Thanks are extended to the San Diego State University Foundation, and to *Robert Carlson* of the Department of Physical Education.

References

Alexander, M.J.L.: The relationship of somatotype and selected anthropometric measures to basketball performance in highly skilled females. Res. Quart. *47:* 575–585 (1976).

Araujo, C.G.S.; Moutinho, M.F.C.: Somatotype and body composition of adolescent Olympic gymnasts. Caderno Artus Med. Desportiva *1:* 39–42 (1978).

Bagnall, K.M.; Kellett, D.W.: A study of potential Olympic swimmers. 1. The starting point. Br. J. Sports Med. *11:* 127–132 (1977).

Carter, J.E.L.: The somatotypes of athletes – a review. Hum. Biol. *42:* 535–569 (1970).

Carter, J.E.L.: Somatotype characteristics of champion athletes; in Novotny, Anthropological Congress Dedicated to Ales Hrdlicka, pp. 241–252 (Academia, Czechoslovak Academy of Sciences, Prague 1971).

Carter, J.E.L.: Somatotype, growth and physical performance; in Vague, Boyer, The regulation of the adipose tissue mass, pp. 259–264 (Excerpta Medica, Amsterdam 1974).

Carter, J.E.L.: The prediction of outstanding athletic ability – the structural perspective. in Landry, Orban, Exercise physiology, pp. 29–42 (Symposia Specialists, Miami 1978a).

Carter, J.E.L.: The somatotypes of Olympic athletes. Paper presented 21st Wld Congr. of Sports Medicine, Brasilia 1978b.

Carter, J.E.L.: The contributions of somatotyping to kinanthropometry; in Ostyn, Beunen,

Simons, Kinanthropometry II, pp. 409–422 (University Park Press, Baltimore 1980a).

Carter, J.E.L.: The Heath-Carter somatotype method (San Diego State University Syllabus Service, San Diego 1980b).

Carter, J.E.L.; Heath, B.H.: Somatotype methodology and kinesiology research. Kinesiol. Rev. *1971:* 10–19.

Carter, J.E.L.; Hebbelinck, M.; Ross, W.D.: Somatotypes of female Olympic rowers. Paper presented 26th Ann. Meet. American College of Sports Medicine, Honolulu 1979.

Chovanova, E.; Zapletalova, L.: Sizes shape and proportion of young basketball players. Paper presented 2nd Int. Symp. on Human Biology (Danube Symposium), Visegrad 1979.

Copley, B.B.: An anthropometric, somatotypological and physiological study of tennis players with special reference to the effects of training; PhD thesis, Johannesburg (1980).

Day, J.A.P.; Duquet, W.; Meerseman, G.: Anthropometry and physique type of female middle and long distance runners, in relation to speciality and level of performance; in Eiben, Growth and development: physique, pp. 385–397 (Akadémiai Kiado, Budapest 1977).

Garay, A.L. de; Levine, L.; Carter, J.E.L. (eds): Genetic and anthropological studies of Olympic athletes (Academic Press, New York 1974).

Duquet, W.; Hebbelinck, M.: Application of the somatotype; attitudinal distance to the study of group and individual somatotype status and relations; in Eiben, Growth and development: physique, pp. 377–384 (Akadémiai Kiado, Budapest 1977).

Falls, H.B.; Humphrey, L.D.: Body type and composition differences between placers and nonplacers in an AIAW Gymnastics Meet. Res. Quart. *49:* 38–43 (1978).

Faulkner, R.A.: Physique characteristics of Canadian figure skaters; MSci thesis, Burnaby (1976).

Guimaraes, A.; Rose, E.H. de: Somatotypes of Brasilian track and field student athletes. Paper presented 21st Wld Congr. in Sports Medicine, Brasilia 1978.

Guimaraes, A.; Rose, E.H. de: Somatotypes of Brazilian student track and field athletes of 1976; in Ostyn, Beunen, Simons, Kinanthropometry, vol. II, pp. 231–238 (University Park Press, Baltimore 1980).

Heath, B.H.: Applying of the Health-Carter somatotype method; in Eiben, Growth and development: physique, pp. 335–347 (Akadémiai Kiado, Budapest 1977).

Heath, B.H.; Carter, J.E.L.: A modified somatotype method. Am. J. Phys. Anthrop. *27:* 57–74 (1967).

Hebbelinck, M.; Carter, L.; Garay, A. de: Body build and somatotype of Olympic swimmers, divers, and water polo players; in Lewillie, Clarys, Swimming, vol. II, pp. 285–305 (University Park Press, Baltimore 1975).

Hirata, K.: Selection of Olympic champions, vol. 1 (Chukyo University, Toyota 1979).

Lebedeff, A.: Body structure of female intercollegiate and junior tennis players; MA thesis, San Diego (1980).

Lowdon, B.J.: The somatotype of international male and female surfboard riders. Aust. J. Sports Med. *12:* 34–39 (1980).

McClure, C.C.: The physiques of professional and amateur women golfers; MA thesis, San Diego (University of Oregon Microcard, PE1027, 1967).

Meleski, B.W.; Shoup, R.F.; Malina, R.M.: Size, physique, and body composition in competitive female swimmers 11 to 20 years of age. Paper presented 49th American Ass. of Physical Anthropologists, Niagara Falls 1980.

Novak, L.P.; Woodward, W.A.; Bestit, C.; Mellerowicz, H.: Working capacity, body composition, and anthropometry of Olympic female athletes. J. Sports Med. phys. Fit. 17: 275–283 (1977).

Perez, B.: Somatotypes of male and female Venezuelan swimmers; in Eiben, Growth and development: physique, pp. 349–355 (Akadémiai Kiado, Budapest 1977).

Perez, B.: Los atletas venezolanos: su tipo fisico, PhD thesis, Caracas (1980).

Rocha, M.L.; Araujo, C.G.S. de; Freitas, J. de; Villasboas, L.F.P.: Antropometria dinamica da Natacao. Revta Ed. Fisica, Brasil 102: 46–54 (1977).

Ross, W.D.; Brown, S.R.; Yu, J.W.; Faulkner, R.A.: Somatotypes of Canadian figure skaters. J. Sports Med. phys. Fit. 17: 195–205 (1977a).

Ross, W.D.; Carter, J.E.L.; Rasmussen, R.L.; Taylor, J.: Anthropometric and photoscopic somatotyping of children; in Shephard, Lavallée, Physical fitness assessment principles, practices and applications, pp. 257–262 (Thomas, Springfield 1978).

Ross, W.D.; Carter, J.E.L.; Roth, K.; Willimczik, K.: Sexual Dimorphism in sport: a comparison of elite male and female athletes by a somatotype I-index, in Eiben, Growth and development: physique, pp. 365–376 (Akadémiai Kiado, Budapest 1977b).

Ross, W.D.; Day, J.A.P.: Physique and performance of young skiers. J. Sports Med. phys. Fit. 12: 30–37 (1972).

Ross, W.D.; Wilson, B.D.: A somatotype dispersion index. Res. Quart. 44: 372–374 (1973).

Salmela, J.H.: Growth patterns of elite French-Canadian female gymnasts. Can. J. appl. Spt Sci. 4: 219–222 (1979).

Shoup, R.F.: Anthropometric and physique characteristics of Black, Mexican-American and White female high school athletes in three sports; MA thesis, Austin (1978).

Sinning, W.E.: Anthropometric estimation of body density, fat, and lean body weight in women gymnasts. Med. Sci. Sports 10: 243–249 (1978).

Sinning, W.E.; Cunningham, L.N.; Racaniello, A.P.; Sholes, J.L.: Body composition and somatotype of male and female Nordic skiers. Res. Quart. 48: 741–749 (1977).

Stepnicka, J.: Typological and motor characteristics of athletes and university students (in Czech) (Charles University, Prague 1972).

Stepnicka, J.: Somatotypes of Bohemian and Moravian youth. Acta facult. med. univ. brunensis, Brno 57: 233–242 (1976a).

Stepnicka, J.: Somatotype, body posture, motor level and motor activity of youth. Acta univ. carolinae gymnica 12: 1–93 (1976b).

Stepnicka, J.: Somatotypes of Czechoslovak athletes; in Eiben, Growth and development: physique, pp. 357–364 (Akadémiai Kiado, Budapest 1977).

Stepnicka, J.; Broda, T.: Somatotypes of young downhill skiers. Teor. Praxe tel. Vych. 25: 166–169 (1977).

Stepnicka, J.; Chytrackova, J.; Kasalicka, V.; Kubrychtova, I.: Somatic preconditions for study of physical education, p. 114 (Univerzita Karlova, Prague 1979a).

Stepnicka, J.; Taborsky, F.; Kasalicka, V.: The somatic prerequisites of women handball players. Teor. Praxe tel. Vych. 27: 746–755 (1979b).

Strong, M.L.: Somatotype and body composition of class I junior female gymnasts; MA thesis, San Diego (1980).

Tanner, J.M.: The physique of the Olympic athlete (Allen & Unwin, London 1964).

Vaccaro, P.; Clarke, D.M.; Wrenn, J.P.: Physiological profiles of elite women basketball players. J. Sports Med. phys. Fit. *19:* 45–54 (1979).

Vivolo, M.A.; Caldeira, S.; Matsudo, V.K.R.: Anthropometric study of the female Japanese National Volleyball team according to the Heath-Carter method. Paper presented 21st Wld Congr. on Sports Medicine, Brasilia 1978.

Westlake, D.J.: Somatotypes of female track and field competitors; MA thesis, San Diego (University of Oregon Microcard, PE1050, 1967).

Dr. J.E. Lindsay Carter, Department of Physical Education, San Diego State University, San Diego, CA 92182 (USA)

Medicine Sport, vol. 15, pp. 117–126 (Karger, Basel 1981)

Influence of Athletic Training on the Maturity Process of Girls

K. Märker

Central Institute of the Sports Medical Service, Kreischa, GDR

Introduction

The interest level of girls and women in sport and the interest in women's sports by the public has increased all over the world. Throughout the centuries deep-rooted prejudices have existed toward female athletic performance based on social values. Until 20 years ago, a large number of physicians had physiological objections based on intuitive traditional attitudes against the adaptability of the female body. However, many girls and women have demonstrated the opposite of their previous medical beliefs by achieving a high degree of athletic performance.

Today, the effects of training on girls is of interest in relation to their athletic performances. It is also a matter of concern with respect to their health and efficiency. Sport during pre-pubescence has been and is still partly opposed. Although clear evidence is available that agility, skill and flexibility reach an optimum during the developmental stages in early childhood and during the first school grades. From 4 to 8 years of age, the child can develop motor coordination and motor skills easily. Therefore, it seems justifiable to begin training with 6- to 7-year-old girls in figure skating, gymnastics and diving under continuous sport medical supervision. During this period, event-specific training elements should never dominate the overall training programme. Instead, attention should be placed upon all-round basic training appropriate to the child's developmental age.

Several authors [*Mayer*, 1952; *Döderlein*, 1956; *Leinzinger*, 1966; *Husslein*, 1975] have consistently warned against too early athletic activities because of the presumed effects on vegetative and generative functions. Since the 1970s researchers throughout the world have supported an early com-

Table I. Mean ages at menarche, standard deviations and ranges in athletes participating in different sport disciplines

Sport disciplines	n	M	SD	Range
Handball	98	13.03	1.00	10.08–15.03
Canoe	32	13.03	1.06	10.08–15.06
Sport students	222	13.06	1.01	11.06–17.00
Volleyball	63	13.07	0.09	11.10–15.03
Swimming	52	13.08	0.11	11.05–15.04
Athletics	102	13.09	1.03	11.03–16.05
Diving	26	14.04	1.06	12.07–17.05
Figure skating	30	15.03	1.09	12.09–19.00
Gymnastics	25	15.04	1.06	13.01–19.03

mencement of training. There has been, however, more speculation about beneficial and harmful effects than there has been evidence of either. Our studies have led to the conclusion that no morphological or functional damages of female genitals are caused by early athletic training. Intensive training during pre-puberty and puberty, however, seems to be accompanied by delayed maturity of the young girls particularly in relation to menarche. However, there was no evidence of increased pathological conditions in female organs – especially in the female genitals – nor restrained femininity or later infertility. Disease or damage that have been diagnosed in single cases of young athletes follow the same statistical pattern objectively analysed as in non-athletic samples. Based upon experience and investigational results, collected over several years, we found that an early beginning of training with girls has generally no detrimental effects on their health status or on their biological development. During the pre-phase of sexual maturity, no safe statements can be made on sex-specific maturity.

While menarche in Central Europe normally occurs between the 11th and 13th year of age, these data are different in female athletes according to their specific sports. The majority of authors reporting data [*Bausenwein,* 1952; *Klaus,* 1954; *Malina* et al., 1978; *Märker,* 1979, 1981; *Prokop,* 1976] found menarche in female athletes occurring somewhat later. *Erdelyi* [1962] found no difference between female athletes and non-athletes while *Ingmann* [1952] *and Åstrand* [1963] observed an earlier occurrence of menarche in swimmers than in non-active women.

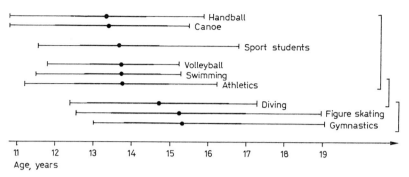

Fig. 1. Mean values (●), standard deviations (heavy lines) and ranges of menarcheal ages of athletes for different sports. Markings at the right side indicate those groups, the mean menarcheal ages of which are not significantly different ($a \leq 1\%$).

Results and Discussion

Investigating 428 female athletes from different sports who trained several times per week from 5 to 15 years, we found a mean menarcheal age of 13.07 years, i.e. 9 months to 16 months later than in non-athletes. Time differences result from reference values of different authors and varying years of studies.

Table I shows menarcheal ages of national or international elite female athletes subdivided according to their events. Looking at the mean values ($\bar{x}$), the standard deviation (SD), and the range of menarcheal ages for each sports, it is clear that there are event-specific differences. The athletes in gymnastics, figure skating and diving had significantly later menarcheal age than other athletes as indicated by the marking at the right side of figure 1 which shows significance at the 1% probability level by the Duncan multiple range test procedure. Our results thus show a menarcheal age similarity within three groups of sport events.

Table II shows the percentage of female athletes who had not experienced menarche by their 15th or 17th year of age, respectively. We can see here, even more obviously, that delayed menarcheal age occurs more in gymnastics, figure skating, and diving than in other sports. The early beginning of intensive athletic activities of all the female athletes suggests event-specific particularities which could be seen as one of the reasons for a different occurrence of menarche. Figure 2 shows that all the female figure skaters, gymnasts, divers and swimmers started training many years before their first menstruation, i.e. during their pre-pubertal phases. The girls'

Table II. Girls without appearance of menarche up to the age cited (in %)

	Menarche: 15 years and later, %	17 years, %
Sport students	3	–
Handball	5	–
Volleyball	6	–
Swimming	8	–
Canoe	12	–
Athletics	18	–
Diving	38	8
Figure skating	44	15
Gymnastics	48	16

ages in these sports ranged from 5.5 to 9 years when they began to engage in athletic exercises. If these ages are related to the mean values of menarche in those 4 sports, a period of 5–10 years on the average is found before menarche occurs.

Swimmers began training 5 years on the average before the occurrence of menarche. However, handball and volleyball were played by the girls only shortly before menarche although they had engaged themselves in ball games at an earlier age. This figure clearly shows that the age to start training differs from one sport to the other. Motor-coordinative skills are easily acquired by girls rather early in their lives. It appears an optimal time for them to learn. To obtain mastery at a later age is often much more difficult. However, endurance or strength oriented sports are started only shortly before menarche. In figure 3 the percentage of female athletes who began athletic activities before menarche is presented. While 100% of the girls in gymnastics, figure skating, and diving started before menarche the percentage was reduced for participants of other sports. There were only 12% in volleyball and 21% in team handball who were actively engaged in these sports before menarche. It becomes quite clear if one considers the high percentage of female swimmers (68%) who had engaged in swimming before menarche that this sport may have a general developmental and fitness impact.

The time of starting training and the duration may be appreciated from figures 2 and 3. No results are presented on the intensity of training. Because nationally and internationally successful female athletes have been investigated, the results are of great value. International athletic perfor-

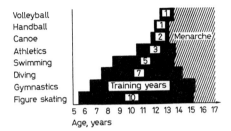

Age, years

Fig. 2. Number of years of training before menarche of female athletes from different sports.

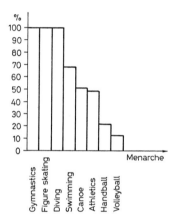

Fig. 3. Female athletes who started training before menarche (%).

mances can only be achieved after several years of systematic and intensive training. Training effects will certainly not become so evident in relation to maturity for participants in recreational activities as with successful competitive female athletes who have much more intensity and duration of training. However, most research shows no harmful effects associated with intensive training regimes. The first menstruation may never be studied in an isolated manner despite the fact that it is a temporarily defined sign of maturation. We have also studied the menstrual relationship of young female athletes and the effect of training on the dynamics of maturation.

As early as 100 years ago, particular attention was concentrated upon menstruation within the field of sport including those various endogenic and exogenic influences. Our interest today is in the same vein but the ques-

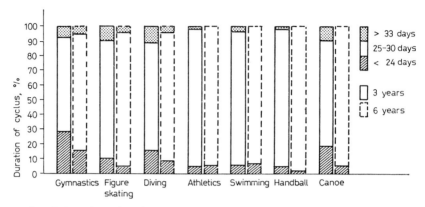

Fig. 4. Duration of cyclus 3 and 6 years after menarche of female athletes from different sports.

tions about menstruation are more pertinent because of the increased emphasis on training of girls and women.

In this research, we have studied the different influences of various sports upon the female athletes' menstruations, 3, 6 and 10 years after menarche. Following a 2- to 3-year regulation from an anovulatoric to an almost bi-phasic cycle, the different subjective and objective parameters are improved in almost all the female athletes' cycles. 3 years after menarche we found cycle durations under 24 days in an average of 8% of the female athletes. After 6 years, this group was reduced to 4.8%. Sport-specific differences were quite obvious. 3 years after menarche, polymenorrhoea was found with 28% of the female gymnasts, 18.8% of canoeists, 15.4% of divers, and 10% of figure skaters. After 6 years these percentages were reduced, as can be seen from figure 4.

A subjective assessment of the intensity of menstrual bleeding was made by the female athletes themselves 3–6 years after menarche. It was clear that 81.3% of them classified the intensity of their menstruation as 'medium' or 'normal' after 3 years, while 88.7% did so after 6 years. An increase of 7.4% after 6 years leads to the conclusion that an intensive athletic activity for several years had no harmful effects upon the intensity of menstruation.

Many authors have stated that athletic training has positive effects upon dysmenorrhoea. Positive effects concerning menstrual problems could be observed immediately after menarche. The effects of training on menstrual pain are important for the maturation of the athlete. Concerning menstru-

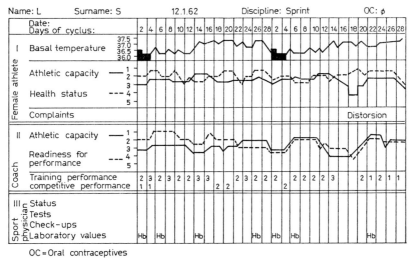

Fig. 5. Cyclogram of a female track and field athlete.

ation, we have included many subjective and objective parameters into a cyclogram (fig. 5) which facilitates the evaluation of performance during the cyclic phases.

The female athlete (I) evaluates her health status and capacity according to the evaluation criteria from 1 to 5 (whereas 1 = very good, 2 = good, 3 = not bad, 4 = bad, 5 = very bad) and registers her basal temperature. The coach (II) assesses her readiness for performance and adds values from training and competition to the self evaluation. The sport physician (III) can include results and laboratory findings into this cyclogram. The investigations are subjective evaluations of the individual's health status during menstruation: the assessment of her athletic capacity; the effects of training and the performance during individual cyclic phases. In addition assessments of the coach, the individuals' physiological performance and the biochemical criteria of the physician were also included as an attempt to evaluate objectively this process.

Despite several years of training during pre-pubescence, no abnormal cycle disturbances appeared which could be attributed to training. However, data in gynaecological literature are rather diverse regarding the frequencies and menstrual disturbances. There are of course menstrual disturbances with female athletes too. But they are much smaller and on an average respond quicker to treatment than with females who are not engaged in

Table III. First parturition of female athletes from different sports (mean ages, standard deviations and ranges)

Sport disciplines	n	Mean age of first parturition M x̄	SD	Range
Volleyball	20	22.02	1.08	18.02–24.08
Canoe	8	22.05	1.10	19.09–24.06
Gymnastics	17	22.08	1.09	19.05–24.09
Rowing	7	23.03	2.07	19.05–27.09
Handball	25	23.04	2.00	19.06–28.07
Skiing	8	23.04	1.07	20.01–24.10
Swimming	18	23.07	1.07	18.07–25.03
Figure skating	6	23.08	2.01	20.01–26.00
Diving	18	23.08	1.11	19.09–28.04
Athletics	107	23.11	1.10	18.03–29.09
Other sports	8	23.07	1.08	20.08–25.10
	242	23.05	1.11	18.02–29.09

sports. Therefore, the effects of athletic training on maturation with girls can only be conclusive when the generative function is confirmed at the highest level of maturity. We have studied the maturation of 242 female athletes after their first parturition. All of these athletes participated in either the GDR, European, World Championships or in the Olympic Games. Among these mothers, the following results include those who were actively training: 18.2% for 6–9 years; 71.5% for 10–14 years; 10.3% for more than 15 years. The average age of their first parturition was 23 years and 5 months. These mothers were either formerly or presently active athletes.

In table III, gymnasts, who have experienced significantly later menarche, show an earlier age of parturition as compared to the other athletes. Figure 6 shows other sport-specific differences. Average values have been included of time of menarche and first parturition of female gymnasts and track-and-field athletes. As a result it becomes obvious that fertility was not impaired despite beginning hard training during early childhood. Those who experienced late menarche appear quickly to reach full maturity. While, generally, female gymnasts gave birth to their first child only after the end of their active athletic career, almost all the other pregnant female athletes stayed active and achieved athletic records even after parturition. For example figure 6 shows that female track-and-field athletes have menarche on

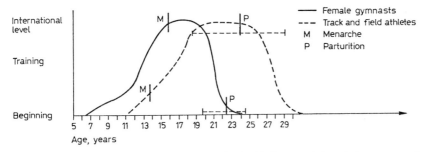

Fig. 6. Beginning of training and individual athletic records in relation to maturity and first parturition of female gymnasts and track and field athletes.

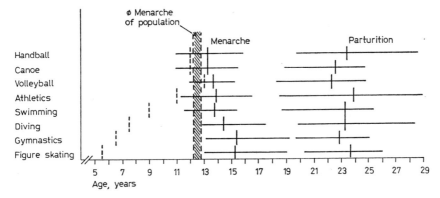

Fig. 7. Beginning of training, mean menarcheal age and range, first parturition and range of athletes from different sports.

the average at the beginning of their athletic career, and have their first child at the climax of their capacity, and continue to remain active.

In figure 7 the occurrence of the important maturity events are shown. There are numerous female athletes known in every country who gave birth to 1, 2 or 3 children during their athletically active career and competed until the end of the third or beginning of fourth life decade.

In conclusion, we have attempted to present the effects on maturation of girls as related to their specific sports. The research includes a large number of nationally and internationally successful female athletes. Although these athletes experienced their menarche on the average later than the other girls, no disadvantages have been found regarding their generative functions based on the data presented on childbirth. The limit of athletic capacity of girls and women has not yet been reached. High athletic performance by many young girl athletes would not be possible by a later beginning of training. The advancing performance in women's sport is also supported by improved social conditions, better health status and enhanced functional efficiency.

Summary

This is a study concerning the effects of maturation on 428 nationally and internationally successful female athletes.

The research begins with their initial interest of their specific sport at an early age and includes their whole athletic period. It was found that these athletes experienced menarche on the average 9–16 months later than the other girls. However, no disadvantage has been found concerning generative functions based on the data presented on childbirth.

References

Åstrand, P.O.; Erikson, B.O.; Nylander, I.; Engström, I.; Karlberg, P.; Saltin, B. and Thoren, C.: Girl swimmers, with special reference to respiratory and circulatory adaptation and gynaecological and psychiatrics aspects. Acta paediat. Suppl. *147* (1963).

Bausenwein, I.: Die deutschen Wettkämpferinnen in Helsinki. Beilage Arzt und Sport. Dt. med. Wschr. *79:* 1526–1532 (1952).

Döderlein, G.: Frau und Leibesübungen; in Arnold, Lehrbuch der Sportmedizin; 1. Aufl., pp. 483–499 (Barth, Leipzig 1956).

Erdelyi, G.J.: Gynecological survey of female athletes. J. Sports Med. phys. Fit. *2:* 174–179 (1962).

Husslein, H.: Frauensport und Menstruationszyklus. Österr. J. Sportmed. *5:* 3–8 (1975).

Ingmann: As cited by Bausenwein, I. (1952).

Klaus, E.J.: Menstrualzyklus, Körperbauform und Sport; in Klaus, Konstitution und Sport (Tries-Verlag, Freiburg/Brsg. 1954).

Leinzinger, D.: Frauenheilkunde und Frauensport auch aus der Sicht der Prophylaxe. Medsche Welt, Stuttg. *17:* 2219–2225 (1966).

Märker, K.: Zur Menarche von Sportlerinnen nach mehrjährigem Training im Kindesalter. Med. Sport *19:* 329–332 (1979).

Märker, K.: Frau und Sport (Barth, Leipzig, in press, 1981).

Malina, R.M.; Spirduso, W.W.; Tate, C.; Baylor, A.M.: Age at menarche and selected menstrual characteristics in athletes at different competitive levels and in different sport. Med. Sci. Sports *10:* 218–222 (1978).

Mayer, A.: Konstitution und Frauenheilkunde. Heilkunst *65:* 1–8 (1952).

Prokop, L.: Einführung in die Sportmedizin (Fischer, Stuttgart 1976).

Dr. med. K. Märker, Central Institute of the Sports Medical Service, DDR-8216 Kreischa (GDR)

Medicine Sport, vol. 15, pp. 127–141 (Karger, Basel 1981)

Physique of Female Athletes - Anthropological and Proportional Analysis

O.G. Eiben

Department of Anthropology, Eötvös Loránd University, Budapest, Hungary

A Question of Kinanthropometry: 'Why is Man of So Large a Size?'

From the many aspects of hominid variation, sexual dimorphism could be said to be the most conspicuous one. Within the female physique, these two distinct types present a wide range of variability. This gamut is more widened by sports and intensive training along with environmental factors. The fact that female athletes display certain kinds of physique which are especially successful in certain events can be considered fact. However, the descriptions of optimum physiques in the single events are, in many instances, incomplete. Therefore, this research paper hopes to provide new data in this field of kinanthropometry.

In order that all these biological endowments and connections can be analyzed, we shall make use of the methods and attitude of kinanthropometry as defined by *Ross* et al. [1980]. While there is abundant anthropometric data and while we know much about the structure of humans, it is not easy to answer the naive, yet profound question, 'Why is man just his actual size?'

It was *Galilei* [1638] who dealt with this question concerning the discussions of animal locomotion. He explains that the small animals are relatively stronger than those of larger body size. He emphasizes that body size was formed in accordance with biological principles and that its development was characteristic of the species. The bones of man (or of an animal) should not be pointlessly big... The body size of the animals can increase in a significant degree, he writes, only if the material of their bones becomes more solid and their capability of resistance gets greater than the usual one; otherwise one has to consider the possibility of a marked thickening of the bones not accompanied by deformation. In his opinion, body enlargement affects all measurements. He presented a bone, the size was about threefold the size of a usual one, yet the animal in question used it just as well as the smaller animals used their bones of smaller sizes.

By now, in the light of the achievements of modern nuclear physics and molecular biology, we see the question somewhat differently. The most valuable part of the human organism is the genetic information which includes the instructions referring to the genetic structure and chemical composition of the organism to further the human growth patterns. All this is recorded in the chromosomes. Consequently, genetic information is fixed not in classically rigid structures but in a molecular system formed as a combination of atoms.

Why then is man so large a size? Why is he just 170 cm tall? Because there is a vast amount of information recorded in each of his cells about what man is. Man is of his actual size because he is clever. Although he does not see the atoms constituting him with the unaided eye, he does understand their operation, and thus the genetic basis of his own existence [*Marx*, 1978].

Even within the biochemical structure of the human body, which already shows certain sexual differences, water deserves special attention. While the details are important and exact specification is an important avenue of needed research in kinanthropometry, we can appreciate gross differences of somewhat typical males and females. About 60% of man's body consists of water (in the case of a body weight of 70 kg this amounts to about 42 kg), only about 55% of the body of a woman is water (in the case of a body weight of 60 kg this is about 33 kg). The difference is not a result of phylogenetic evolution but is related to the higher fat content (near 30%) of the female body. There is also a difference in the distribution of water. Namely, the extracellular water content was 15% with each of the two sexes; however, in men intracellular water amounted to 45% and only 40% in women. The water content of the body also changes with age, as this is generally known (in men it decreases to about 54% by the age of 60–80 years, at the same time to about 46% in women).

Water content is closely connected with the specific gravity. In the human body the specific gravity of the bone is 1.56, which includes the soft parts of 1.06 while that of the adipose tissue was 0.94. The specific gravity of the lean body mass (LBM) was about 1.10. If we assume a linear dependence between the specific gravity and fat content of the body, a 10% increase of the fat content would result in a decrease of specific gravity by 0.02. The fat content of the body of a normally fed men would be 18–20%, and his specific gravity would be about 1.06.

From the viewpoint of sports, the fat content of the body may be even more important. The literature on LBM is rather large and often inadequate; therefore, the author merely refers to it here. Of the brief data mentioned, the significance of composition is clearly discernible.

Purpose of the Survey

The morphological differences of female athletes can be demonstrated by comparing several different body measurements and proportional characteristics. The different groups of female athletes are well distinguished on the basis of their physique within a population. Research has shown that there is a connection between physique and being successful in sports [*Eiben*, 1972].

The existence of these adequate constitutional endowments in gifted young individuals may be one of the biological bases of a successful sport enthusiast. (We do know, however, that a recorder-accomplishment has many other components, too.) As we analyze by kinanthropometry the physique of the outstanding female athletes, we defined the desired body size, shape, proportions and composition of each kind of sport. These 'optimal' types of physique are what we attempted to discover in the gifted young athletes.

By *physique*, we mean the morphological constitution of an individual, which is formed by the manifestation of genetic endowment and the result of adaptation to environmental effects [*Eiben,* 1972].

Procedure: Material and Methods

To analyze the physique of different kinds of outstanding European and Hungarian female athletes, the author has investigated the following groups:

Female track-and-field athletes were surveyed at the VIIIth European Athletic Championship organized in Budapest in 1966. The 125 female athletes came from 13 countries and their ages varied between 15 and 36, yielding a mean of 23.8 years [*Eiben*, 1972].

Female ballplayers were investigated in Budapest in the 1970s: (a) *volleyball players*, 25 members of the Hungarian national team, age 16–33, mean 20.3 years; (b) *basketball players*, 30 members of the Hungarian national team, age 17–31, mean 21.4 years;

(c) *handball players*, 29 members of the Hungarian national team, age 19–32, mean 23.4 years.

Female fencers, 26 members of the Hungarian national team, age 18–34, mean 23.0 years [*Eiben*, 1972].

Female table tennis players, 31 outstanding European players coming from 9 countries, whose ages varied between 16 and 38, the mean was 21.2 years [*Eiben and Eiben*, 1979].

In the course of the examinations a full anthropometric program using the methods of *Martin and Saller* [1957–1966] and *Tanner* et al. [1969] was performed, internationally accepted in anthropometry. A valid instrument for the analysis of the proportions is *Ross and Wilson's* [1974] unisex human phantom as a metaphorical model. The analysis of body composition is served by the recently introduced metric methods which, besides the measurements of circumference of the extremities, refer to separate muscle circumference. The cross-sectional area and the muscle area of the extremities, respectively, strive to exclude subcutaneous fat from the measurements of the extremities [*Jeliffe*, 1966]. Finally, the samples were elaborated by applying the method of the generalized component analysis.

Findings

The body measurements of the female track-and-field athletes have been published by *Eiben* [1972], and their proportions were reported by *Eiben* et al. [1976]. Their physique was analyzed by factor analysis [*Eiben and Csébfalvi*, 1977].

Table I shows the female ballplayers' body measurements and proportional data [*Eiben*, 1980]. The factor-analysis study of *Eiben and Csébfalvi* [1977] includes some data of the volleyball and basketball groups. The body measurements and proportional data of the female fencers and the female table tennis players were also published earlier [*Eiben*, 1972; *Eiben and Eiben*, 1979]. Based on these previous studies, and completed with some new data, the author attempted to give a detailed description on the physique of the various female athletes.

Female Track-and-Field-Athletes

Sprinters. Among the runners, the body measurements of the sprinters (n = 22) were inferior to the means of all the surveyed female track-and-field athletes in each anthropometric character. They were small in stature ($\bar{x}$ = 165.3 cm), and their weight was considered light. Their small stature was due mainly to their short trunk. Their lower extremities, especially their thighs were relatively long as compared with the trunk. Their development in width was moderate; however, their shoulder width was proportionally

Table I. Body measurements of the female ballplayers

Body measurements	x̄	s	sx̄	W	z
(a) Volleyball players (n = 25)					
Stature	174.75	4.81	1.39	168.0–185.7	–
Sitting height	90.48	3.35	0.67	82.0– 96.0	0.47
Suprasternal height	141.84	4.43	0.89	134.0–151.0	1.35
Symphysis height	92.20	3.03	0.61	88.0– 99.0	1.76
Shoulder (acromion) height	142.72	4.40	0.88	134.0–152.0	1.32
Elbow (radiale) height	111.08	3.40	0.68	104.0–117.0	1.28
Wrist (stylion) height	86.72	3.14	0.63	80.0– 92.0	1.54
Finger (dactylion) height	66.60	2.92	0.58	60.0– 71.0	1.35
Length of the upper extremity	76.58	4.98	1.44	71.8– 91.1	–1.28
Height of the ant. sup. iliac spine					
(lower extremity length)	99.28	3.53	0.71	93.0–108.0	1.17
Knee (tibiale) height	47.32	2.23	0.45	43.0– 52.0	0.60
Ankle (sphyrion) height	7.76	1.20	0.24	7.0– 9.0	–0.04
Head height	20.36	1.12	0.22	18.0– 23.0	–0.35
Shoulder (biacromial) width	39.33	1.38	0.40	37.3– 41.7	–0.76
Bideltoid width	41.92	1.47	0.29	38.0– 46.0	–0.19
Chest breadth	26.36	1.35	0.27	23.0– 29.0	–0.49
Chest depth	15.72	1.14	0.23	14.0– 18.0	–0.98
Bi-iliocristal width	29.64	1.32	0.26	27.0– 33.0	0.91
Bitrochanter width	35.08	1.31	0.38	33.6– 37.5	0.01
Chest circumference	84.17	2.81	0.81	80.5– 89.0	–1.82
Abdomen circumference	82.47	4.12	0.82	73.0– 93.0	1.27
Trochanter circumference	93.42	4.26	1.23	84.2–100.8	–1.40
Upper arm circumference relaxed	24.67	1.38	0.40	22.2– 26.7	–1.70
Upper arm circumference contracted	25.24	1.24	0.25	23.0– 28.0	–1.47
Upper arm muscle circumference	19.48	1.69	0.34	17.0– 24.0	–
Forearm circumference	22.83	0.71	0.02	21.8– 24.0	–1.76
Wrist circumference	15.32	0.81	0.16	14.0– 17.0	–0.86
Thigh circumference	56.00	3.04	0.88	51.5– 60.0	–0.64
Calf circumference	35.50	1.36	0.39	33.0– 38.4	–0.90
Calf muscle circumference	22.16	1.80	0.36	29.0– 36.0	–
Ankle circumference	21.96	1.21	0.24	20.0– 24.0	0.63
Bicondylar humerus, mm	64.60	2.73	0.55	60.0– 70.0	0.44
Bicondylar femur, mm	97.03	4.02	0.80	89.0–106.0	0.93
Wrist width, mm	52.36	2.20	0.44	49.0– 57.0	0.99
Biceps skinfold, mm	5.92	1.89	0.38	3.0– 10.0	–0.96
Triceps skinfold, mm	15.48	4.13	0.83	8.0– 24.0	0.11
Subscapula skinfold, mm	12.64	3.27	0.65	7.0– 19.0	–0.83
Suprailiaca skinfold, mm	12.56	4.84	0.97	4.0– 22.0	–0.56
Umbilical skinfold, mm	14.16	5.24	1.05	8.0– 25.0	–1.40

Table I. continued

Body measurements	x̄	s	sx̄	W	z
Calf (medial) skinfold, mm	11.00	2.48	0.50	7.0– 16.0	–1.01
Upper arm area, cm²	47.00	4.58	0.92	39.0– 57.0	–
Upper arm muscle area, cm²	30.52	5.07	1.01	24.0– 45.0	–
Calf area, cm²	101.72	8.97	1.80	85.0–117.0	–
Calf muscle area, cm²	83.24	9.50	1.90	69.0–101.0	–
Weight, kg	64.28	5.33	1.07	52.1– 74.4	0.17
(b) Basketball players (n = 30)					
Stature	176.63	6.71	1.23	162.1–187.2	–
Sitting height	91.43	3.27	0.60	85.0– 98.0	–0.58
Suprasternal height	144.10	7.19	1.31	132.0–153.0	0.11
Symphysis height	93.53	4.27	0.78	84.0–101.0	0.72
Shoulder (acromion) height	146.20	5.98	1.09	132.0–156.0	0.29
Elbow (radiale) height	114.10	4.94	0.90	102.0–123.0	0.51
Wrist (stylion) height	89.20	4.60	0.84	78.0– 99.0	0.80
Finger (dactylion) height	69.10	3.58	0.65	61.0– 76.0	0.82
Length of the upper extremity	75.80	3.50	0.64	67.5– 81.7	–0.86
Height of the ant. sup. iliac spine (lower extremity length)	99.80	4.94	0.90	90.0–107.0	–0.02
Knee (tibiale) height	48.47	2.33	0.43	44.0– 53.0	–0.10
Ankle (sphyrion) height	7.70	0.92	0.17	6.0– 9.0	–0.61
Head height	21.50	2.32	0.42	20.0– 23.0	–0.53
Shoulder (biacromial) width	38.90	1.79	0.33	34.0– 42.0	–0.38
Bideltoid width	42.80	2.37	0.43	38.0– 47.0	–0.93
Chest breadth	26.67	1.88	0.34	24.0– 31.0	–1.27
Chest depth	18.37	1.48	0.27	16.0– 21.0	0.15
Bi-iliocristal width	30.00	1.72	0.31	27.0– 34.0	0.05
Bitrochanter width	34.20	2.04	0.38	31.0– 39.0	0.14
Chest circumference	86.07	4.72	0.86	76.0– 94.3	–0.99
Abdomen circumference	82.33	5.47	1.09	73.0– 96.0	0.07
Trochanter circumference	98.03	5.47	1.00	90.0–108.5	0.10
Upper arm circumference relaxed	24.60	1.80	0.33	21.0– 28.0	–1.42
Upper arm circumference contracted	26.30	1.97	0.36	22.0– 30.0	–1.71
Upper arm muscle circumference	19.73	1.26	0.23	18.0– 23.0	–
Forearm circumference	23.90	1.32	0.25	22.0– 27.0	–1.34
Wrist circumference	15.50	0.91	0.17	14.0– 17.0	–1.96
Thigh circumference	57.60	2.90	0.54	52.0– 65.0	0.08
Calf circumference	36.50	2.10	0.39	31.0– 40.0	–0.48
Calf muscle circumference	32.83	1.90	0.35	29.0– 37.0	–
Ankle circumference	23.03	1.79	0.33	21.0– 27.0	0.37
Bicondylar humerus, mm	64.00	3.70	0.74	58.0– 71.0	–0.89

Table I. continued

Body measurements	x̄	s	sx̄	W	z
Bicondylar femur, mm	97.10	5.92	1.18	87.0–106.0	–0.33
Wrist width, mm	52.70	2.83	0.52	48.0– 58.0	–0.07
Biceps skinfold, mm	8.03	2.99	0.55	4.0– 16.0	–0.13
Triceps skinfold, mm	14.87	4.94	0.90	7.0– 27.0	–0.24
Subscapula skinfold, mm	11.97	3.43	0.63	7.0– 21.0	–1.12
Suprailiaca skinfold, mm	15.70	5.27	0.96	6.0– 35.0	–0.06
Umbilical skinfold, mm	18.83	5.67	1.03	7.0– 31.0	–0.94
Calf (medial) skinfold, mm	11.70	3.76	0.69	7.0– 22.0	–1.01
Upper arm area, cm²	47.73	6.84	1.25	35.0– 60.0	–
Upper arm muscle area, cm²	31.30	4.22	0.77	25.0– 41.0	–
Calf area, cm²	105.97	11.75	2.15	81.0–129.0	–
Calf muscle area, cm²	86.40	10.17	1.86	76.0–108.0	–
Weight, kg	67.18	8.47	1.55	54.0– 82.1	0.02
(c) Handball players (n = 29)					
Stature	168.48	5.29	0.98	156.5–182.2	–
Sitting height	88.69	2.38	0.44	83.0– 93.0	–0.17
Suprasternal height	136.69	4.86	0.90	126.0–150.0	0.08
Symphysis height	87.00	3.91	0.73	78.0– 98.0	0.29
Shoulder (acromion) height	138.62	5.21	0.97	127.0–153.0	0.24
Elbow (radiale) height	107.69	4.12	0.77	100.0–120.0	0.38
Wrist (stylion) height	84.97	3.22	0.60	79.0– 94.0	0.86
Finger (dactylion) height	66.52	2.83	0.53	61.0– 74.0	1.09
Length of the upper extremity	72.06	3.24	0.59	66.0– 77.6	–0.87
Height of the ant. sup. iliac spine (lower extremity length)	92.86	3.47	0.65	84.0–105.0	–0.43
Knee (tibiale) height	46.00	2.28	0.42	39.0– 44.0	–0.11
Ankle (sphyrion) height	7.41	0.58	0.11	7.0– 9.0	–0.51
Head height	20.86	0.92	0.17	20.0– 23.0	–0.09
Shoulder (biacromial) width	39.10	1.31	0.24	36.0– 42.0	0.76
Bideltoid width	43.03	1.61	0.30	40.0– 46.0	0.08
Chest breadth	28.03	1.15	0.21	26.0– 31.0	0.31
Chest depth	18.72	1.42	0.26	16.0– 21.0	1.09
Bi-iliocristal width	29.21	1.50	0.28	26.0– 32.0	0.46
Bitrochanter width	33.30	1.58	0.29	30.9– 37.0	0.55
Chest circumference	87.20	4.10	0.76	82.5–101.2	0.06
Abdomen circumference	81.83	3.42	0.64	75.1– 90.2	0.49
Trochanter circumference	94.52	4.44	0.83	87.3–105.4	0.14
Upper arm circumference relaxed	25.55	1.80	0.33	22.9– 30.6	–0.47
Upper arm circumference contracted	27.48	2.59	0.48	25.0– 37.0	–0.64
Upper arm muscle circumference	20.45	1.38	0.26	18.0– 24.0	–

Table I. continued

Body measurements	x̄	s	sx̄	W	z
Forearm circumference	24.23	1.33	0.25	21.6– 27.5	–0.47
Wrist circumference	15.38	0.75	0.14	13.0– 17.0	–1.03
Thigh circumference	58.10	3.49	0.65	53.0– 66.1	0.68
Calf circumference	36.20	2.84	0.52	31.8– 42.9	0.58
Calf muscle circumference	32.17	2.58	0.48	27.0– 37.0	–
Ankle circumference	22.79	1.61	0.30	20.0– 28.0	1.07
Bicondylar humerus, mm	64.20	3.84	0.74	57.0– 73.0	1.10
Bicondylar femur, mm	98.30	5.92	1.13	88.0–111.0	0.95
Wrist width, mm	52.00	2.60	0.48	45.0– 57.0	0.64
Biceps skinfold, mm	9.83	3.59	0.67	3.0– 16.0	0.99
Triceps skinfold, mm	16.17	4.29	0.80	10.0– 25.0	0.23
Subscapula skinfold, mm	14.07	4.45	0.83	7.0– 26.0	–0.58
Suprailiaca skinfold, mm	15.62	5.40	1.00	7.0– 24.0	0.10
Umbilical skinfold, mm	15.93	5.85	1.09	4.0– 26.0	–1.19
Calf (medial) skinfold, mm	13.24	3.81	0.71	8.0– 21.0	–0.55
Upper arm area, cm²	51.48	8.14	1.51	42.0– 62.0	–
Upper arm muscle area, cm²	33.28	4.41	0.82	27.0– 44.0	–
Calf area, cm²	105.03	16.32	3.03	77.0–147.0	–
Calf muscle area, cm²	82.62	13.08	2.43	71.0–111.0	–
Weight, kg	64.90	7.01	1.30	55.5– 81.5	0.06

wide (biacromial width, z=0.73). Their upper extremities were less muscular, but their lower limbs, especially their lower legs, were proportionally strong with well-developed muscles (calf circumference, z=0.22). According to our statistical procedure of factor analysis, sprinters were small (factor 1: magnitude), their slenderness (factor 2: procerity) as well as the development of their muscles (factor 3: firmity) were medium, and they had a boyish physique (factor 4: femininity).

Hurdlers. Actually, female hurdlers (n=12) are strong and muscular sprinters. Their stature was nearly identical with the sprinters' stature; however, their trunk was somewhat longer and stronger (biacromial width, z=0.95), and their lower extremities were relatively short (x̄=55.6%, z=–0.36). Regarding the proportions of their lower extremities, long legs and shorter thighs were characteristic of the hurdlers. Their upper extremities were slender, not very muscular; however, their lower extremities were muscular, especially their lower legs (calf circumference, $\bar{x} = 35.8$ cm, $z = 0.66$). The hurdlers were corpusculent (in factor 1), and their procerity and firmity was medium. As a result, their physique was manish.

Middle-Distance Runners. The body of the female middle-distance runners (n = 26) was the most linear, the most slender one of all the measured female track-and-field athletes. They were the smallest in stature ($\bar{x} = 164.8$ cm) and the lightest. Also their Kaup morphological index as well as their body surface were the smallest of all. Their trunk was the longest ($\bar{x} = 47.6$ cm) and the narrowest; however, their chest depth (sagittal diameter) was an exception in this respect ($\bar{x} = 18.4$ cm, $z = 1.11$). Their chest circumference ($\bar{x} = 86.9$ cm) was the widest among all the female runners. Their muscles were not massive, almost gracile. Their physique was medium in the first three factors and resembled a manish form.

Long Jumpers. Between the two groups of jumpers, the female long jumpers (n = 9) were somewhat smaller in stature ($\bar{x} = 170.8$ cm). Their trunk was longer and their lower extremities were shorter than those of the high jumpers. Their lower legs were very long ($\bar{x} = 41.2$ cm), being the longest of all examined groups. Their width development was remarkable (biacromial width, $z = 0.60$; bitrochanter width, $z = 0.64$; chest depth, $z = 0.58$). However, their extremities were not very muscular. Their magnitude was medium, in procerity they were not slender, in firmity they were strong, and they had a boyish physique.

High Jumpers. The high jumpers (n = 13) were taller in stature ($\bar{x} = 172.8$ cm). Their trunk was relatively short, it was not very wide, but relatively slender. Their lower extremities were rather long ($\bar{x} = 93.6$ cm, $z = 0.00$), just like their thighs ($\bar{x} = 46.1$ cm). Their width development and the development of the muscles in their extremities were moderate. In this respect, they come close to the mean of all surveyed female track-and-field athletes: usually, they were decidedly superior to those of the runners; however, they remained below those of the throwers. In the two factors, in magnitude and in procerity they were medium, in firmity they were strong, their physique was boyish.

Shot Putters. The female throwers generally were tall and muscular. The Kaup index of the female shot putters (n = 11) was the highest among all female track-and-field athletes. They weighed much and their stature ($\bar{x} =$ 170.2 cm) was tall. Their long trunk was accompanied with long lower extremities. Similarly their thighs were very long, but their lower legs were relatively short. Again, their upper extremities were only slightly longer than the average of all female track-and-field athletes. They excelled with a marked width development, especially their shoulder girdle was highly developed with a biacromial width of $\bar{x} = 40.8$ cm ($z = 1.42$) and bideltoid breadth of $\bar{x} = 46.5$ cm ($z = 1.25$). Their trunk was proportionally wide (chest breadth, $z = 1.10$; chest depth, $z = 2.08$; chest circumference, $z = 1.89$; bitrochanter width, $z = 1.65$). The shot putters had the most muscular extremities among all the measured female athletes, especially the muscles of their thighs were well developed (thigh circumference, $\bar{x} = 64.6$ cm, $z = 2.07$). Their body was corpusculent, heavy, in firmity they were medium, and they had a boyish physique.

Discus Throwers. The female discus throwers ($n = 8$) were the tallest and most highly developed female athletes. Their stature was $\bar{x} = 174.9$ cm, none of them lower than 165 cm. They weighed heaviest among all female athletes (weight, $\bar{x} = 81.5$ kg). Similarly, the length of both their trunk and lower extremities were the greatest. Their lower legs were relatively long, and their thighs relatively short. Their upper extremities were long and strong. Characteristically, they displayed the longest span of $\bar{x} = 182.9$ cm. They were ahead also as to width measurements, especially their shoulder girdle was well-developed (biacromial width, $\bar{x} = 41.7$ cm, $z = 1.40$; bideltoid breadth, $\bar{x} = 47.4$ cm, $z = 1.07$). Their trunk was proportionally wide. The muscles of their extremities were highly developed, proportionally great, yet they surpassed shot putters only in forearm circumference. The magnitude of their body was great, in procerity they were thick, in firmity medium, and they were boyish.

Javelin Throwers. The female javelin throwers ($n = 8$) weighed least among all female throwers, and their stature was scarcely taller than that of the shot putters. The relative length of the proximal parts dominated in their extremities. As compared with the other female throwers, the development of their width and that of the muscles of their extremities was moderate. Their shoulder girdle, however, was well-developed, and their lower extremities were proportionally strong. The magnitude of their body was great, in procerity they were medium, in firmity they excelled with thin muscles, and their physique was boyish.

Pentathlonists. The data of the female pentathlonists (n = 16), who pur-
sued each athletic event, agreed in most characters with those typical of all
female track-and-field athletes, or deviated from them to a minimum in the
positive direction. Their shoulder girdle was proportionally well-developed
(biacromial width, $\bar{x} = 39.2$ cm, $z = 0.72$), as compared with their pelvic
girdle (bitrochanteric width, $z = 0.18$), as well as their muscular extremities,
especially their lower ones, should be emphasized here. In magnitude their
body was very great, in procerity they were slender, in firmity medium, and
they had a boyish physique.

Female Ballplayers

Another opportunity of comparison is provided by three groups of
female ballplayers.

Volleyball Players (table I a). In the female volleyball players (n = 25)
a linear build of the body was especially apparent. They were tall in stature
($\bar{x} = 174.8$ cm), with proportionally long lower extremities (lower extremity
length, $z = 1.17$). Their trunk was relatively wide, but not robust, their pelvic
girdle was proportionally large (bi-iliocristal width, $z = 0.91$). Only the muscularity of their upper arms can be pointed out. Their mean somatotype was
3.72, 3.96, 3.12. Their body in magnitude was very great, in procerity they
were not slender, in firmity they were relatively strong, and they had a
womanish physique. There was a conspicuous connection between their
not robust (however, also not gracile) body build and the nature of the
volleyball game which does not need too many place-changing movements.

Basketball Players (table I b). The female basketball players (n = 30)
were taller in stature ($\bar{x} = 176.6$ cm) with a narrow trunk that was more
robust. Their extremities were linear, but more muscular. Because of this,
they were more fit for the somewhat harder team games involving much
running and sudden changes of position, whereas in the hand-to-hand attempts at ball control, a physique rather similar to that of the female track-
and-field athletes has a significant function. Their mean somatotype was
3.75, 3.80, 3.47. Their body was corpusculent, and they were very slender
and strong. Their physique was girlish.

Handball Players (table I c). The female handball players (n = 29) were
the shortest in stature ($\bar{x} = 170.18$ cm, just like the unisex phantom) among
the three ballplayers groups. They were the most muscular, with wide

shoulders and a relatively robust trunk. Their chest depth was proportionally wide (z = 1.09, cf. middle-distance runners). They had relatively long and very muscular upper extremities. Their mean somatotype was 4.50, 4.09, 2.17. Their body mass, both in endomorphy and mesomorphy, was related to a strong team game, as in the case of men. Their physique was boyish.

Female Fencers

As compared with the surveyed female athletes, the female fencers (n = 26) were of a low stature ($\bar{x}$ = 164.7 cm), they were even shorter than the female runners. Their relatively short lower extremities accounted for that. All their length measurements – also including their sitting height and span – were shorter by about 1 cm than those of the runners. Their width development was moderate. Their biacromial width ($\bar{x}$ = 36.9 cm) was smaller than that of any groups of the female track-and-field athletes measured. Their bideltoid breadth ($\bar{x}$ = 40.5 cm) comes near only to that of the middle-distance runners. The structure of their chest reminded us of that of the runners: it was relatively narrow (chest breadth, $\bar{x}$ = 25.9 cm) and deep (chest depth, $\bar{x}$ = 17.9 cm), their chest circumference was medium ($\bar{x}$ = 85.9 cm). Their waist and trochanter were narrow, just like those of the runners. Their abdomen and trochanter circumferences were, however, greater. As to muscularity, their extremities generally agreed with those of the runners and jumpers, only their thighs were exceptions, being very muscular with a thigh circumference of $\bar{x}$ = 57.8 cm. Their weight ($\bar{x}$ = 60.4 kg) was less than the average of all measured female track-and-field athletes; however, it surpassed that of the runners. Their body build in magnitude was very small, in procerity very slender, in firmity relatively strong, and they had a girlish physique.

Female Table Tennis Players

The female table tennis players (n = 31) were moderately tall (stature, $\bar{x}$ = 163.6 cm) and not too linear. Their trunk can be characterized by not narrow shoulders, but deep chest and round hips. Their extremities were slim and not too muscular, the upper ones were proportionally short. Furthermore, their extremities had thin bones and a greater quantity of subcutaneous fat than expected. Their mean somatotype, 4.5, 3.3, 2.7, was shifted towards meso-endomorphy. Their body build in magnitude was very small, in procerity very slender, in firmity they excelled with their thin muscles and they had a girlish physique.

Discussion

The relationship of the physique and athletic movements of the female track-and-field athletes was well-investigated and it was quite obvious.

Two other very clear examples were given in this paper. One of them is the case of a deep chest in all female athletes who need a great stamina. At 'endurance-events' like middle-distance running or fencing or table tennis we can find a great value of antero-posterior chest diameter, which is connected with the function of the lung. The intensive ventilation supposes or, better said, requires a deep chest. The build of the chest in antero-posterior direction seems to be more important from a physiological point of view than the transversal one.

Another example is served by the three groups of female ballplayers. There is a very typical line of variability according to characteristic movements of each game.

The volleyball players play in a relatively small space, they do not need to run, and to strive with body against body, their game may be characterized rather by skill than many place changes. They were linear and relatively gracile compared to the other ballplayers.

The basketball players had to perform as quick runners, i.e. they had to change their place permanently; their physique must be fit for this kind of team game. Handball play was the hardest female ballgame, with continuous running and wild body contacts. The handball players, who excelled with their very deep chest, were the most muscular, the most robust ballplayers.

These examples demonstrated very well the connection of *structure* and *function*. The essential relationship of these two has held the attention of researchers since research began. It can be considered a basic principle of biology that each structure becomes suitable for performing a definite function by the very peculiarity of its construction. In the majority of cases, it is easy to perceive the connection of strucure and function. For example the relationships between the dense vascularity of the parenchymal organs, of the liver, the kidney, the heart and their considerable oxygen demand, and further between the curvatures and the resilience or flexibility of the spinal column as well as the spatial arrangement of the elements of bone tissue and mechanical load are conspicuous.

Until now, anthropology examined its subject mostly and preponderantly statically. The greater part of our attainments has been inspired by morphology. However, one must not lose sight of the circumstance that structure and function are sides of the same material system, which possibly should be taken simultaneously into consideration. Yet these two aspects of the phenomenon are manifested not only by their inseparability but by a relative independence of each other as well. A given structure or parts of it may change without any alteration ensuing in the functional characteristic of that structure. Yet it has also been reported that the biological systems of identical structures worked functionally differently.

Our future objective should be to search for the functional meaning of the given structures at the time they are recognized. We should try to connect the functions more intensively with the structural characteristics.

Naturally, this is not a new endeavor in biology, yet it becomes increasingly significant today. Relatively soon, after the macroscopic analysis of structure and function, came the microscopic examination (cellular and then intracellular analysis). Intercellular structure could be experimentally influenced as early as the 1930s. However, on the intercellular level the way was opened only after a significant advance in genetics. With the development of ultrastructure research, as well as with the biophysical and biochemical methods, the relationships between the structural and functional characteristics of the living organisms are being examined today on the level of the protein molecule. The electron microscopic examination of the ultrastructure led to the recognition of new functions [*Eiben*, 1979]. All these ideas could give new views to our research in the near future, and help further progress of kinanthropometry.

Summary

The author sketches the importance of the female athletes' size, shape, and body proportions from the view of kinanthropometry. He investigated different groups of outstanding European and Hungarian female athletes (such as track-and-field, ballplayers, fencers and table tennis players). A detailed anthropometric program was used and analyzed by factor analysis. Based on the results, a detailed kinanthropometric description of the individual physique of the various athletic groups is presented. Also, a discussion concerning the relationship of the athlete's anthropometric structure and function is presented.

References

Eiben, O.G.: The physique of woman athletes (The Hungarian Scientific Council for Physical Education, Budapest 1972).

Eiben, O.G.: Functional biotypology in Hungary (Opening Lecture at the 2nd Int. Symp. on Human Biology, Visegrád 1979).

Eiben, O.G.: Recent data on variability in physique: some aspects of proportionality; in Ostyn, Beunen, Simons, Kinanthropometry, vol. II, pp. 69–77 (University Park Press, Baltimore 1980).

Eiben, O.G.; Csébfalvi, K.: Recent data to the analysis of the variations of physique; in Eiben, Growth and development: Physique. Symp. Biol. Hung., vol. 20, pp. 417–430 (Akadémiai Kiadó, Budapest 1977).

Eiben, O.G.; Eiben, E.: The physique of European table-tennis players. Coll. Anthropol. 3: 67–76 (1979).

Eiben, O.G.; Ross, W.D.; Christensen, W.; Faulkner, R.A.: Proportionally characteristics of female athletes. Anthrop. Közl. 20: 55–67 (1976).

Galilei, G.: Discorsi e dimostrazioni matematiche, intorno a due nuove scienze, attenenti alla mecanica e i movimenti locali (Impression anastaltique, Leida, 1638).

Jeliffe, D.B.: The assessment of the nutritional status of the community. WHO Monogr. Ser., vol. 53 (WHO, Genève 1966).

Martin, R.; Saller, K.: Lehrbuch der Anthropologie I–IV. (G. Fischer Verlag, Stuttgart 1957–1966).

Marx, G.: Életrevaló atomok (Resourceful atoms). (Akadémiai Kiadó, Budapest 1978).

Ross, W.D.; Drinkwater, D.T.; Baily, DMA.; Marshall, G.R.; Leahy, R.M.: Kinanthropometry: traditions and new perspectives; in Ostyn, Beunen, Simons, Kinanthropometry, vol. II, pp. 3–27 (University Park Press, Baltimore 1980).

Ross, W.D.; Wilson, N.C.: A stratagem for proportional growth assessment; in Borms, Hebbelinck, Children and exercise. Acta paediat. belg. suppl., pp. 169–182 (1974).

Tanner, J.M.; Hiernaux, J.; Jarman, S.: Growth and physique studies; in Weiner, J.S.; Lourie, F.A. (Eds.): Human Biology. A guide to field methods. IBP Handbook 9 (Blackwell, Oxford-Edinbourgh 1969).

Dr. O.G. Eiben, Puskin u. 3, H-1088 Budapest (Hungary)

Medicine Sport, vol. 15, pp. 142–149 (Karger, Basel 1981)

Asymmetry of Limb Circumferences in Female Athletes

E. Zaharieva

Department of Sports Medicine and Sports Massage,
Higher Institute of Physical Culture, Sofia, Bulgaria

The study of morphological asymmetry of limbs in female athletes is of great interest with regard to the principle of harmony in body-build, on the one hand, and in relation to physical fitness and performance, on the other hand. In the available literature, no data concerning morphological asymmetry in women athletes can be found. Most investigations focus on functional asymmetry from the viewpoint of age development [*Skopakov*, 1954, 1959] or age change in physical fitness [*Potzeluev*, 1960; *Alipieva*, 1972] and partly in respect to some kind of sports [*Ilin*, 1961; *Tulilov*, 1969; *Ahlborg* et al., 1975; *Oyster*, 1979].

The purpose of our investigation was to study morphological asymmetry in limb circumferences of female athletes in order to discover the effect of sports on the physical development of women. We investigated athletes practicing those kinds of sports which lead to the development of asymmetry in limbs and also sports in which physical exercises engage the extremities equally. 1,634 women and 1,915 men engaged in 14 kinds of sports were examined, although the women were additionally compared to competitors in modern gymnastics (96 women). We also took into consideration a part of the anthropometric investigations on a large scale on the physical development of elite Bulgarian and foreign athletes carried out by the collaborators of the department.

In the present paper we examine: (1) character of the morphological asymmetry of limb circumferences in female athletes; (2) morphological asymmetry depending on the kind of sports; (3) differences in morphological asymmetry in men and women engaged in sports.

Table I. Number of subjects according to the kind of sports

Kind of sports	Women	Men
Gymnastics	279	250
Track-and-field events	92	217
Swimming	107	91
Rowing	199	148
Canoe – kayak	20	40
Diving	15	13
Skiing	34	57
Tennis	21	40
Fencing	54	126
Acrobatics	49	52
Judo	81	94
Basketball	317	368
Volleyball	255	312
Handball	111	107
Modern gymnastics	96	
Totals	1,730	1,915

Procedure

Measurements of 5 limb circumferences were taken: upper arm, contracted and relaxed; forearm (data were obtained from 1,111 women and 1,080 men); thigh, and leg. The measurements were made with a tape measure according to the following method. The upper arm circumference was measured, m. biceps brachii and m. brachialis being contracted to the maximum, at its most bulging part (the forearm in horizontal position, and a right angle between upper arm and forearm). Immediately after that measurement the circumference of the upper arm in a relaxed state was measured. The tape measure was held at the same level on the horizontal plane with elbow extended and the extremity relaxed. Then, the forearm circumference was measured with the tape measure placed horizontally at its largest part (the extremity relaxed). Thigh circumference was measured with the subject's feet straddled at shoulder width, body weight being equally distributed on both legs. The tape measure was placed immediately below the gluteal fold in the horizontal plane. Leg circumference was taken in the same position of the body with the tape measure placed horizontally in the region of the greatest protuberance of m. triceps surae.

Under asymmetry we understand an increase in the size of a certain limb circumference in comparison to the same circumference of the other limb when the difference is over 0.3 cm [*Shapovalov* et al., 1976].

The age of most of the subjects ranged from 17 to 28 years, and the length of time of their sports practice ranged from 6 to 20 years. In order to establish the statistical sig-

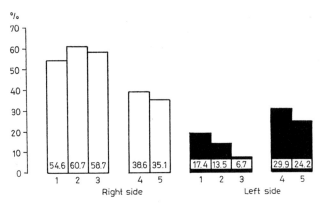

Fig. 1. Percentage of occurrence of asymmetry in female athletes: (1) upper arm relaxed; (2) upper arm contracted; (3) forearm; (4) thigh; (5) leg.

nificance of the differences, we used the t-test. A difference was considered significant when $t = 2.5$ or $p = 0.01$. The number of subjects engaged in different kinds of sports is given in table I.

Results

Morphological asymmetry of the limb circumferences in female athletes is mainly a right-sided one and it is observed more often in the upper than in the lower extremities (fig. 1). Right-sided asymmetry in the upper limbs was found, in most of the female athletes, with the upper arm contracted (60.7%) and in the lower limbs, for thigh circumference (38.6%). Asymmetry of the left upper extremities was more rare in female athletes. For the upper arm (contracted) it was observed in only 13.5% of the female athletes. Relatively more frequently, we observed left-sided asymmetry of thighs (in 29.9% of the female athletes).

Morphological asymmetry of limb circumferences in men is of the same character as in women (fig. 2). However, asymmetry in men was more frequently observed than in women but the differences were not significant ($p = 0.05$) at the proposed level. The magnitude of morphological asymmetry in most of the female athletes varied between the very low values of 0.5–1 cm (fig. 3). Asymmetry over 1 cm was observed more frequently in the upper arm contracted (24.5%) and thigh circumferences (19.8%). A greater percentage of cases with morphological changes in limb circumfer-

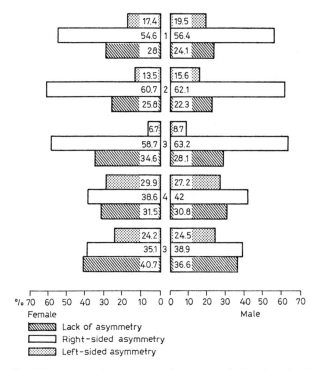

Fig. 2. Percentage of occurrence of asymmetry in female and male sportsmen. Numbers 1–5 as in figure 1.

ences over 1 cm was observed in men and the difference with females was significant (p = 0.01).

The effect of the kind of sports practiced on morphological asymmetry of extremities in women athletes was studied in 15 sports and 1,730 competitors. Right-sided asymmetry of the upper extremities was most frequently found in the upper arm contracted and in the forearm. This measurement was present mostly (between 87.5 and 70.6%) in female athletes engaged in tennis, fencing, basketball, handball, track, skiing and volleyball (fig. 4). Most often right-sided asymmetry of thighs was observed in women competitors engaged in handball (60%), fencing (59.3%) and modern gymnastics (53.1%) (fig. 5) and of legs in female competitors engaged in modern gymnastics (50%) and kayak (50%).

A relatively high proportion of left-sided asymmetry of thighs (fig. 5) was found in female skiers (76.5%) and tennis players (57.1%). Depending on the ski event, left-sided asymmetry of thighs was observed for downhill

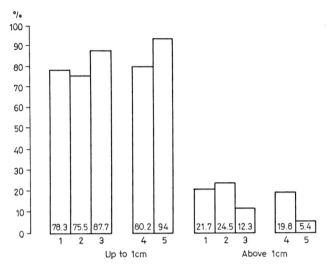

Fig. 3. Percentage of occurrence in female athletes of right-sided asymmetry, up to 1 cm and above 1 cm. Number 1–5 as in figure 1.

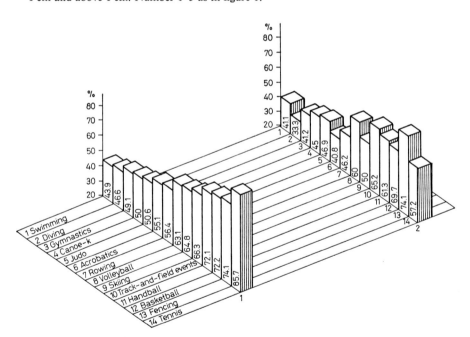

Fig. 4. Percentage of occurrence of right-sided asymmetry in upper limbs in female athletes in relation to the kind of sports practiced: (1) upper arm contracted; (2) upper arm relaxed.

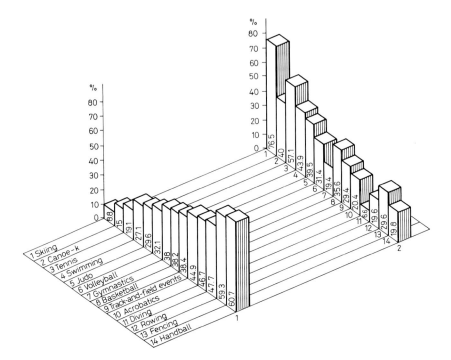

Fig. 5. Percentage of occurrence of asymmetry in female athletes in relation to the kind of sport: (1) right-sided asymmetry; (2) left-sided asymmetry.

and slalom ski events in 64.7% of the competitors, and for cross-country skiing in 88.2%.

Asymmetry of limb circumferences was not found mainly in women competitors in gymnastics, diving, etc. The absence of asymmetry in the forearms of competitors in gymnastics (70.1%), rowing (55.7%), acrobatics (49%) could be explained by the equal engagement of the forearms in these sports events.

The extent of asymmetry depending on the kind of sports practiced showed changes of more than 1 cm most frequently in the contracted upper arm circumference and in the thigh circumference of women competitors in basketball, handball, fencing, rowing.

The effect of the kind of sports practiced on limb asymmetry in women athletes is of a similar character as in men engaged in the same kinds of sports.

Discussion

A great variety was observed in the morphological asymmetry of limb circumferences in female athletes as a result of the different physical exercises and techniques used in sports. In women athletes, asymmetry was found both in the upper and in the lower limbs. Most often, however, a right-sided asymmetry was noted, predominantly in the circumferences of the large muscle groups of the upper arm and thighs. The morphological changes were small and in the range of 0.5–1 cm. The character of the asymmetry in women athletes was almost the same as in men. In the latter, asymmetry in the circumferences of the forearm and leg muscles was observed much more often, and the values of the asymmetry were higher – over 1 cm.

The morphological asymmetry of limb circumferences was found to be highly dependent on the kind of sports practiced. In those kinds of sports where conditions exist for unilateral effort of the limbs, asymmetry in women was more frequently established. In sports where there exist conditions for equal engagement of the opposite limbs, asymmetry was observed in a smaller percentage of the subjects. The character of the asymmetry in male and female athletes was not the same in all sports.

Conclusions

(1) The morphological asymmetry of limb circumferences in female athletes is mainly a right-sided one and is more frequently observed in the upper limbs (upper arm and forearm contracted). Left-sided asymmetry is rarely noted in female athletes and mostly in the lower limbs, specifically in the thigh circumference. (2) Lack of asymmetry is more often observed in the leg circumference. (3) The magnitude of morphological changes in limb asymmetry is in the range of 0.5–1 cm in the majority of the women athletes. (4) Relationships were found between morphological asymmetry and the kind of sports practiced. Asymmetry in limb circumferences is established more often in women competitors engaged in tennis, fencing, sports games, skiing, and to a lesser degree in gymnastics, diving, swimming and acrobatics. (5) Comparative investigations on male and female athletes show that asymmetry does not differ in character, but only in frequency and magnitund.

Summary

Morphological asymmetry of limb circumferences was studied in order to establish the effect of sports on the physical development of women. Measurements were taken from 1,730 women engaged in 15 sports and from 1,915 men engaged in 14 sports. Morphological asymmetry in women athletes was found to be mainly right-sided and most frequently in the upper extremities. The values of asymmetry were mostly up to 1 cm.

Relationships were noted between asymmetry and the kind of sports practiced. The comparison of data obtained from male athletes did not point to differences in the character of asymmetry, but only in its frequency and extent.

References

Ahlborg, G.; Hagenfeldt, L.; Wahren, J.: Substrate utilization by the inactive leg during one leg or arm exercise. J. appl. Physiol. *39:* 718–723 (1975).

Alipieva, V.: Za funktzionalnata assimetria na gornite krajnitzi v nachalnata uchilishtna vazrast. Vapr. na fiz. kult. *6:* 351–359 (1972).

Ilin, I.P.: Vlijanie mnogoletnej adnastaronnej trenirovki na stepen vyrajennosti funktzionalnoj assimetrii. Teorija i praktika fizich. kult. *3:* 200–203 (1961).

Oyster, N.: Effects of a heavy resistance weight training program on college women athletes. J. Sports Med. phys. Fit. *19* (1979).

Potzeluev, A.A.: Assimetrija dvijenij. Teorija i praktika fizich. kult. *7:* 496–498 (1960).

Shopakov, V.; Lipvinov, V.; Dzyak, G.; Harchenko, V.: Methodicheskiye rekomendacii po ocenka fizicheskogo razvitiya sportsmenov, p. 19 (Dnepropetrovsk 1976).

Skapovalov, H.: Razvitie na predpochitanieto na po-chestata upotreba na edinija ot krajnitzite. Izvestija na Instituta za fizichesko vaspitanie i uchilishtna higiena, pp. 219–247 (Izdanie na Bulgarska akademija na naukite, Sofia 1959).

Skopakov, H.: Razlikite mejdu krajnitzite pri desnjatzi i levatzi. Nauchni trudove na Meditzinskata akademija, pp. 69–90 (Darjavno izdatelstvo Nauka i izkustvo, Sofia 1954).

Tulilov, I.: Kam vaprossa za funktzionalnata assimetria na dolnite krajnitzi. Vapr. na fiz. kult. *3* (1969).

Dr. E. Zaharieva, Higher Institute of Physical Culture,
Tina Kirkova Str. 1, 1000 Sofia (Bulgaria)

Medicine Sport, vol. 15, pp. 150–156 (Karger, Basel 1981)

Some Differences Between Men and Women in Various Factors which Determine Swimming Performance

H. Vervaecke, U. Persyn

Katholieke Universiteit Leuven, Instituut Lichamelijke Opleiding,
Unit 'Aquatics', Heverlee, Belgium

Introduction

In nearly all sports the absolute performance values of males are higher than those of females. However, in swimming the differences are less marked than in most other sports, thus women can be said to perform relatively better than men in this area.

Significant differences between the sexes have been clearly identified in anthropometric, strength and flexibility data [*Mosterd*, 1961; *Kukushkin*, 1963; *Hirata*, 1966; *Tittel and Wutscherk*, 1972; *Kunze* et al., 1976; *de Garay* et al., 1974; *Bulgakova*, 1978], but the relevance of these measurements for swimming speed in the four strokes and in the various stroke patterns has not been investigated.

It was decided therefore to study the above parameters and relate them to swimming speed in the various strokes and thus identify specific performance attributes in women which enable them to perform relatively better at swimming compared to men than they do at other sports.

Procedure

47 Belgian national elite swimmers of each sex aged 10–22 years were assessed by a battery of 44 anthropometric, 10 flexibility, 7 isometric-strength and 90 time-space style parameters, the selection of which was primarily based on film-observation of top-level swimmers by *Persyn* [1974].

The anthropometric measurements enabled us to identify height, endomorphy, mesomorphy and ectomorphy (calculated by the Heath-Carter technique), relative hand surface and foot surface (relative to the maximal horizontal cross-section of the chest); relative

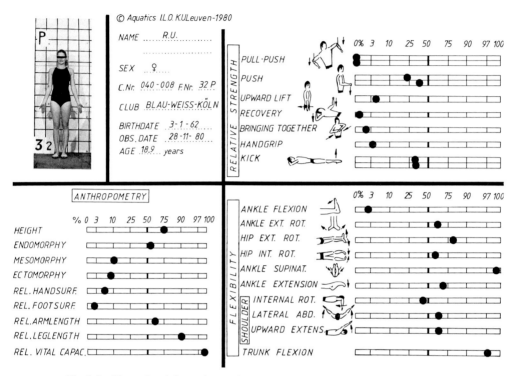

Fig. 1. Profile card mainly used to rank anthropometric, flexibility and strength parameters in the Belgian population of competitive swimmers. Percentile scales were
constructed. The result obtained for each individual measurement is presented as follows:
where the marker (●) covers the 75th percentile, 25% score better than this subject.

arm length and leg length (relative to standing height), and relative vital capacity (relative
to the body weight) (fig. 1). The flexibility measurements and isometric strength tests
[Vervaecke and Persyn, 1979] are also shown in figure 1.

Basic speed (over 10 m) was measured in each of the four strokes i.e. front crawl,
backstroke, butterfly and breaststroke, in total stroke and in pulling or kicking only.
These speed tests were filmed simultaneously from both side view under water (16 mm
Bolex EL camera, 32 frames/s) and front view, above and under water (super 8 mm Canon
cameras, 24 frames/s); and the films analyzed for technical efficiency of each subject at all
phases of all strokes [Persyn, 1974].

All data were processed by SPSS computer programs [Nie et al., 1970]. Variance
analysis was used to identify differences between age groups ($p \leq 0.05$).

The most relevant of the various data were presented on profile cards pertaining to
the Belgian population of competitive swimmers per age and sex [Persyn et al., 1979]
(fig. 1) to aid immediate practical use of the information. Standard score profiles for

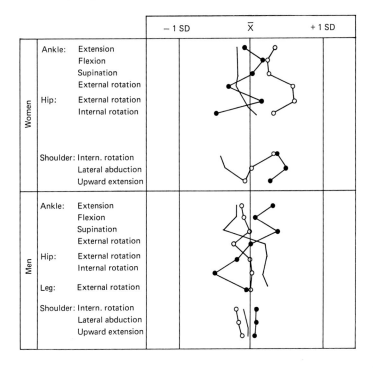

		− 1 SD	X̄	+ 1 SD

Women

Ankle: Extension
           Flexion
           Supination
           External rotation

Hip: External rotation
         Internal rotation

Shoulder: Intern. rotation
           Lateral abduction
           Upward extension

Men

Ankle: Extension
           Flexion
           Supination
           External rotation

Hip: External rotation
         Internal rotation

Leg: External rotation

Shoulder: Intern. rotation
           Lateral abduction
           Upward extension

Fig. 2. Standard score profile of some flexibility results of three age groups of women and men Belgian elite swimmers (means and standard deviations derived from data of all swimmers). ○ = 16–22 years (n women = 12) (n men = 18); line only = 13–15.9 years (n women = 21) (n men = 14); ● = 10–12.9 years (n women = 14) (n men = 15).

strength and flexibility were constructed for three age groups within each sex (fig. 2, 3) and models were constructed to compare the swimmers with the normal Belgian population [*Simons* et al., 1980] and also with another elite group of swimmers (fig. 4) [*Tittel and Wutscherk*, 1972].

Results

As compared to the male swimmers, the females demonstrated significantly higher endomorphy and lower mesomorphy values (p < 0.05), thus confirming the findings of *de Garay* et al. [1974] on top-level competitors at the Mexico Olympic Games (table I).

The women showed significantly lower relative values of surfaces of hand and foot (p < 0.01), of arm and leg length (p < 0.05) and of vital ca-

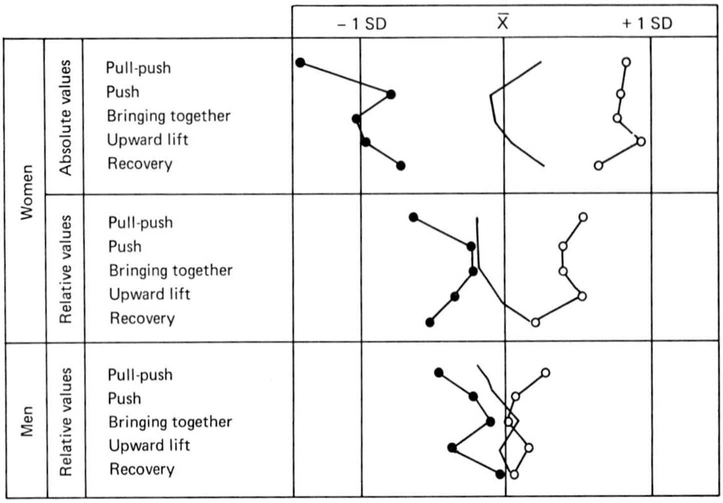

			− 1 SD	X̄	+ 1 SD	
Women	Absolute values	Pull-push Push Bringing together Upward lift Recovery				
	Relative values	Pull-push Push Bringing together Upward lift Recovery				
Men	Relative values	Pull-push Push Bringing together Upward lift Recovery				

Fig. 3. Standard score profile of some strength results of three age groups of women and men Belgian elite swimmers (means and standard deviations derived from data of all swimmers). Data and signs are the same as in Fig. 2.

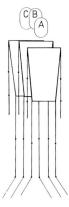

Fig. 4. Models of three different populations (15 years old): A = Belgian average; B = Belgian elite swimmer; C = GDR elite swimmer.

pacity (p < 0.01). These findings supported those obtained by *Skipka* [1979] on top level swimmers.

The floating capacity of the women, as inferred from the respective densities, was slightly better than that of the men (D = 1.0661, 1.0727, respectively), a result in keeping with those obtained by *Szabö and Szabö* [1969] and *Bulgakova* [1978].

Table I. Anthropometric differences between male and female Belgian swimmers

	Male (n=47)		Female (n=47)		Differ-ences	t-Test probability level
	x̄	SD	x̄	SD	%	
Relative hand surface	0.230	0.021	0.210	0.022	8.69	**
Relative foot surface	0.267	0.028	0.239	0.029	10.48	**
Relative arm length	44.78	1.62	42.85	1.47	4.28	*
Relative leg length	48.54	1.37	46.58	1.00	4.08	*
Relative vital capacity	71.07	8.05	64.92	7.36	8.65	**
Endomorphy	2.03	0.64	3.29	0.88		*
Mesomorphy	4.32	1.20	3.42	0.81		*
Ectomorphy	4.25	0.82	3.80	0.61		

* $p < 0.05$; ** $p < 0.01$.

The women demonstrated greater flexibility in all joints, particularly at the ankle ($p < 5\%$), though the difference was not significant at the shoulder. The men always showed higher values on relative strength tests (11%, $p < 1\%$).

Analysis of the films showed that although men had greater relative hand surface, arm length and strength, their hand positions in the pull phase were less effective than those of the women, and their slipping of the hand through the water was much more pronounced (11%). Women would thus appear to better utilize their more limited somatic and motor potential by operating at a higher level of competency.

The finding in the women's group of a correlation of $r = 0.77$ between the speed obtained in 400 m kicking and total stroke would appear to indicate a greater relative importance of kicking within the female sample, which is in agreement with the finding that the men always performed better in pulling; though the specific reason behind this greater facility for kicking has not been identified as yet.

Comparison of the female swimmers in the three age groups (fig. 2) revealed a number of differences. The oldest group had higher densities, lower ectomorphy values and smaller relative hand and foot surfaces and leg lengths. The oldest group was more flexible than the other groups, especially at the ankle and their within group variance was lowest for this parameter. The comparison of the general anthropometric data of the middle group of swimmers (both male and female) to the Belgian population average

and to data from the best swimmers found in that age group in East Germany [*Tittel and Wutscherk*, 1972] or Russia [*Bulgakova*, 1978] revealed a close proximity between the two swimming groups (fig. 4).

Discussion and Conclusion

Despite the limited number of subjects and the relatively low performance level of the Belgian swimmers on an international basis, it would appear that there are a number of factors in part responsible for the improved relative performance of women in the sport of swimming. In addition to the existence of slightly better capacity to float, the two major factors identified would appear to be better joint flexibility and more appropriate stroke mechanics, i.e. greater technical proficiency. Just why women are more competent technically is not readily apparent. The answer may lie in a greater reliance on strength in the men to the ongoing detriment of technique, or may stem from a particular relationship between muscle bulk and joint mobility.

The results of the intergroup comparisons on the women would appear to give some backing to this point. The oldest group was strongest in all force data – both absolute and relative (fig. 3), and least flexible in the shoulder joint, about which we would expect the greatest muscle build-up. Flexibility would appear to be less affected in the lower body by increasing strength or age, since the oldest group also demonstrated the greatest ankle flexibility (fig. 2). A suggested explanation for this was that there was a drop out of the less talented, and therefore less flexible swimmers with age, which, if true, would emphasize the lower shoulder flexibility in the oldest group and further point to some interrelationship between muscle build-up and joint mobility. Further study along these lines is obviously warranted in the quest for performance improving factors.

Summary

Anthropometric, flexibility and strength measures were taken on 47 male and 47 female Belgian swimmers and swim test films were analyzed to assess whether women, who perform relatively better than men in swimming compared with other sports, possess special performance attributes specific to this sport. Factors identified which may support this theory included better floating capacity, greater joint flexibility and more appropriate stroke mechanics.

References

Bulgakova, H.: The selection and preparation of young swimmers (in Russian) (Moscow, 1978).

Garay, A. de; Levine, L.; Carter, J.E.L.: Genetic and anthropological studies of Olympic athletes (Academic Press, New York 1974).

Hirata, K.: Physique and age of Tokyo Olympic champions. J. Sports Med. phys. Fit. 6: 207–222 (1966).

Kukushkin, G.: The peculiarities of the physical development of sportsmen of various specializations. Medicina dello Sport 3: 701–708 (1963).

Kunze, D.; Hughes, P.; Tanner, J.: Anthropometrische Untersuchungen an Sportlern der XX. Olympischen Spiele 1972 in München (Anthropometric research on athletes of the Olympic Games from München); in Jungman, Sportwissenschaftliche Untersuchungen während der XX. Olympischen Spiele, München 1972, pp. 33–56 (Demeter, Gräfeling 1976).

Mosterd, W.: Stuwkrachtmeting en slaganalyse bij getrainde zwemmers (Measuring propulsive force and analysing the stroke of trained swimmers) (Schotanus & Jens, Utrecht 1961).

Nie, N.; Hull, C.; Jenkins, J.; Steinbrenner, K.; Bent, D.: Statistical package for the social sciences (McGraw-Hill, New York 1970).

Persyn, U.: Technisch-hydrodynamische benadering van de bewegende mens in het water (Technical-hydrodynamic approach of human motion in water), pp. 5–136 (Hermes, Leuven 1974).

Persyn, U.; Vervaecke, H.; Hoeven, R.; Daly, D.: Technical evaluation and orientation for skill in sprinting for competitive swimmers. Int. Congr. P.E., Quebec 1979 (in press).

Simons, J.; Beunen, G.; Ostyn, M.; Renson, R.; Gerven, D. van; Witte, L. de: The Leuven Boys Growth Study: norms and profile charts; in Ostyn, Beunen, Simons, Kinanthropometry, vol. II, pp. 263–288 (University Park Press, Baltimore 1980).

Skipka, W.: Anthropometrische Probleme im Schwimmsport (Anthropometric problems in swimmers). Schwimmtrainer 9/10: 31–34 (1979).

Szabö, J.; Szabö, Z.: Anthropometrische und spezifische Gewichtsmessungen an ausländischen und hiesigen Teilnehmern des Internationalen Schwimmwettkampfes in Budapest (Anthropometric and specific weight measurements within competitors of the international event in Budapest). Sportarzt Sportmed. 20: 152–157 (1969).

Tittel, K.; Wutscherk, H.: Sportanthropometrie (Barth, Leipzig 1972).

Vervaecke, H.; Persyn, U.: Effectiveness of the breaststroke leg movement in relation to selected time-space, anthropometric, flexibility, and force data, in Terauds, Bedingfield, Swimming, vol. III, pp. 320–328 (University Park Press, Baltimore 1979).

H. Vervaecke, Katholieke Universiteit Leuven, Instituut Lichamelijke Opleiding, Unit 'Aquatics', Heverlee (Belgium)

Medicine Sport, vol. 15, pp. 157–167 (Karger, Basel 1981)

Body Composition and Somatotype Characteristics of Sportswomen

P. Bale

Chelsea School of Human Movement, Brighton Polytechnic,
Eastbourne, England

Introduction

Many studies, particularly during the past 15 years, have revealed a positive relationship between body build and performance, in which top-class sportsmen have a high muscular component [*Behnke and Wilmore*, 1974; *Carter*, 1970; *de Garay* et al., 1974; *Gayton*, 1975; *Hirata*, 1966; *Leek*, 1969; *Lewis*, 1966; *Maas*, 1974; *Sinning* et al., 1978; *Tanner*, 1964]. Although fewer in number, similar studies have been published relating physique, particularly somatotype, and performance of women athletes [*Alexander*, 1976; *Brown and Wilmore*, 1971; *Falls and Humphrey*, 1978; *Hay and Watson*, 1970; *Johnston and Watson*, 1968; *Malina* et al., 1971; *Sinning* et al., 1978].

Methods

The moderate relationships obtained between physical performance variables such as balance, agility, endurance and strength and body build in specialist women physical education students [*Bale*, 1979, 1980] encouraged the author to examine the relationship between body build and different types of sports performance. Anthropometric measurements such as height, weight, skinfolds, circumferences, and bone widths were used to estimate somatotype and body composition in the following groups of sportswomen: International field hockey players (n=15); The British Colleges women's cross-country champions (n=6); members of the Polytechnic champions women's basketball team (n=7); members of the College modern educational gymnastic display team (n=7); members of the College swimming team (n=9).

The gymnastic and swimming group consisted exclusively of specialist physical education students who represent the Polytechnic in these two activities. The cross-country runners and basketball players, though they had PE students in their teams, also

included students from other faculties of the college. In the hockey group there were students from other colleges and other parts of England. The ages of the sportswomen ranged from late teens to early twenties.

In addition to these groups, *McNaught-Davis* supplied anthropometric data taken from groups of top-class women cyclists, track-and-field athletes and ballet dancers. The ballet dancers were younger than the other groups. Their mean age was 17.5 with an age range of 15.9–19.5 years.

The somatotype was assessed using the Parnell M4 technique [*Parnell*, 1958]. Body density, percent fat, absolute fat and lean body weight were calculated from the sum of four skinfolds, using the regression equation of *Durnin and Rahaman* [1967]. Body density is estimated from the logarithm of the sum of the biceps, triceps, subscapula and supra-iliac skinfolds. Logarithmic instead of absolute values are used since the relationship of skinfolds to density is curvilinear [*Durnin and Rahaman*, 1967; *Durnin and Womersley*, 1974]. Percent fat is estimated from body density using the Siri equation [*Siri*, 1956].

$$\left(\frac{4.95}{D} - 4.5 \right) \times 100.$$

The equations are considered by their authors to have a high reliability and accurately estimate body composition when compared with direct methods such as body volumetry, hydrostatic weighing or body potassium analysis.

A multivariate analysis of variance and canonical analysis was carried out in which linear combinations of all the original 19 variables were made to find which best revealed the differences between the five groups of sportswomen.

The earlier study of cyclists, track-and-field athletes and ballet dancers was mainly concerned with an investigation into the differences in leg volume, so there was insufficient data to calculate somatotype or to include these subjects in the statistical analysis. However, body composition was assessed in the same way as above from those anthropometric measurements available.

Results

The mean scores and standard deviations of the anthropometric measurements and the somatotypes of the sportswomen are presented in table I. In addition, the distribution of somatotypes is illustrated in the somatochart (fig. 1). Heights, weights, ponderal indices and the mean scores of body composition are presented in tables II and III.

The multivariate analysis of variance indicated significant differences in physique between the five sports groups as shown by Bartlett's V value [*Tatsuoka*, 1971]. The X^2 of 110.9 (76 d.f.) pointed at a significance at the 1% level. To investigate further how and where the groups differed canonical variables, which serve as linear discriminant functions [*Maxwell*, 1968], were calculated. Four canonical variables were isolated, the first of which was also significant at the 1% level (X^2 56.1 with 22 d.f.).

Table I. The mean scores and standard deviations of the anthropometric measures and somatotype of sportswomen

Sports group	Height cm	Weight kg	Skinfolds, mm					Condyles, cm		Girths, cm		Ponderal index	Endo-morphy	Meso-morphy	Ecto-morphy
			biceps	triceps	scapula	iliac	thigh	humerus	femur	biceps	calf				
Hockey players (15)															
Mean	165.2	61.5	7.90	14.22	8.99	8.13	20.44	6.19	8.88	27.31	35.71	12.57	3.5	4.1	2.6
SD	5.6	4.5	2.7	4.1	1.6	2.0	3.7	0.36	0.34	1.6	1.9	0.40	0.55	0.59	0.79
Cross-country runners (6)															
Mean	160.0	48.7	7.15	10.07	7.75	5.73	14.28	6.22	7.85	23.08	31.53	13.60	2.8	3.0	4.8
SD	8.9	4.1	3.4	3.3	2.6	0.64	2.7	0.94	0.97	0.81	1.3	0.27	0.61	0.32	0.82
Basketball players (7)															
Mean	171.5	64.8	9.37	12.99	10.33	8.92	22.58	6.24	8.73	27.11	34.64	12.74	3.7	3.4	3.3
SD	2.9	4.3	1.4	3.3	1.5	3.1	2.2	0.23	0.32	1.9	1.6	0.68	0.49	0.79	0.76
Swimming team (9)															
Mean	163.1	58.7	9.18	13.78	10.38	7.57	21.33	6.02	8.96	27.31	35.87	12.81	3.6	4.0	2.7
SD	7.4	7.7	3.1	5.1	2.7	2.3	4.9	0.38	0.36	2.0	1.6	0.40	0.68	0.71	0.83
Gymnasts team (7)															
Mean	162.3	58.2	8.23	14.20	9.93	8.92	22.20	5.95	8.78	27.02	34.91	12.73	3.5	3.9	2.9
SD	4.7	7.2	2.8	2.8	3.6	3.1	5.9	0.46	0.47	2.7	2.7	0.37	0.58	0.69	1.0
Total (45)															
Mean	164.6	59.17	8.35	13.36	9.47	7.78	20.4	6.13	8.71	26.64	34.83	12.8	3.58	3.89	2.85
SD	6.77	7.2	2.7	4.0	2.4	2.2	4.7	0.47	0.59	2.3	2.3	0.53	0.63	0.65	1.20

The number of subjects tested in each activity is shown in parentheses.

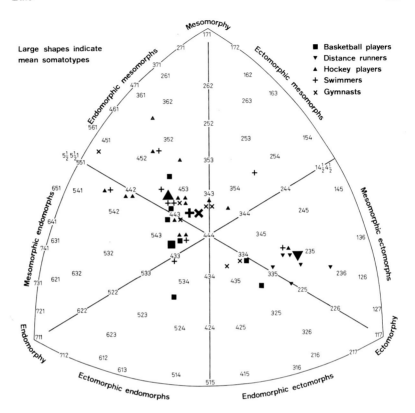

Fig. 1. Distribution of somatotypes of five different groups of sportswomen.

    The graphical representation of the five groups of sportswomen using
the first two canonical variables is given in figure 2. It clearly demonstrates
the discriminating power of the canonical variable analysis. The group means
of the two variables are shown in table IV. The first canonical variable
(horizontal axis) separated the subjects into four distinct groups: the hockey
players; the basketball players; the swimmers and gymnasts; and the cross-
country runners, mainly on the basis of a combination of weight and height,
percent fat, femur bone width and biceps girth. The hockey players tended
to score high on these variables and the cross-country runners low. The
second variable (vertical axis) separates the subjects into three groups: the
hockey players, swimmers, and gymnasts; the cross-country runners; and

Table II. The height, weight and ponderal indices of the sports groups

Sports group	Height cm	Range	Weight kg	Range	Ponderal index	Range
Hockey players (15)	165.2	156.4–171.7	61.5	54.2–69.2	12.6	12.0–13.3
Cross-country runners (6)	160.0	148.6–170.5	48.7	40.6–52.2	13.6	13.2–14.0
Basketball players (7)	171.5	170.4–176.3	64.8	64.0–70.1	12.7	12.4–13.4
Swimming team (9)	163.1	152.4–172.0	58.7	48.8–69.6	12.8	12.2–13.5
Gymnastic display team (7)	162.3	157.0–168.9	58.2	50.0–73.0	12.7	12.7–13.3
Cyclists (11)	161.6	151.6–166.9	58.0	50.0–70.6	12.7	12.2–13.3
Athletes (11)	168.4	159.0–180.0	60.56	51.3–71.1	13.0	12.4–13.4
Ballet dancers (21)	161.1	150.1–168.5	44.7	34.5–55.8	13.8	12.7–14.6
Physical education students (53)	166.3	153.2–180.0	61.3	48.8–80.2	12.9	11.3–13.7

The number of subjects tested in each activity is shown in parentheses. The scores of a group of women physical education students have also been included for purposes of comparison.

basketball players. It is explained mainly by a combination of high measures of triceps and iliac skinfolds and mesomorphy on the hockey players, swimmers, and gymnasts in comparison with the cross-country runners and basketball players.

Discussion

As a group the somatotypes of the sportswomen indicate that they are less endomorphic and more mesomorphic than non-athletic women of a similar age. The somatotypes of most women lie below the ectomorphic axis in the endomorphic sectors of the somatochart [*Sheldon* et al., 1954; *Parnell*, 1958]. The mean somatotype of the women students measured by *Parnell* [1958], for example, was 4.5–3.5–3 compared with the mean of 3.5–4–3 for these sportswomen. As a group, the sportswomen have a mean percent fat of 22.6% which is less than that reported both for non-athletic women by *Durnin and Womersley* [1974] and a group of physical education students measured by the author (table III). All three studies used the same

Table III. The mean scores and standard deviations of body composition measurements of sportswomen

Sports group	Density	% fat	Absolute fat	LBW
Hockey players (15)				
Mean	1.0468	22.90	14.19	47.34
SD	0.005	2.3	2.1	3.5
Cross-country runners (6)				
Mean	1.0557	18.90	9.03	39.95
SD	0.004	1.8	0.88	3.8
Basketball players (7)				
Mean	1.0466	23.0	14.98	50.39
SD	0.008	1.0	1.4	3.5
Swimming team (9)				
Mean	1.0440	23.93	14.19	44.14
SD	0.009	4.0	3.8	3.7
Gymnasts (7)				
Mean	1.0461	23.24	13.93	44.4
SD	0.008	3.5	4.0	3.3
Cyclists (11)				
Mean	1.0431	24.57	14.47	43.4
SD	0.006	2.8	2.9	3.8
Athletes (11)				
Mean	1.0499	21.49	13.10	47.5
SD	0.008	3.8	3.8	3.6
Ballet dancers (21)				
Mean	1.0484	22.16	9.99	34.7
SD	0.005	2.2	1.8	3.8
Physical education students (53)				
Mean	1.0450	23.56	14.61	46.72
SD	0.008	3.82	3.96	4.3

The mean scores of a group of women physical education students have also been included for purposes of comparison.

estimate of body composition. The density of 1.0473 g/cm³ and absolute body fat of 13.6 kg compares very closely to *Brown and Jones'* [1977] group I, which consisted of physical education students who were training for competition in a variety of sports at national and international level including swimming, hockey, basketball, netball and athletics. Although *Brown and Jones* [1977] found no differences between groups in distribution of fat with reference to the amount of activity, there was a wide range of individual variation within each of their activity groups.

The cross-country runners are noteworthy for the narrow range of variation in their physical parameters. Their somatotypes are largely mesomorphic ectomorphs. These girls were significantly lower in percent fat than the other sportswomen, indicating that female endurance runners, like their male counterparts, have a light frame, one that is best suited to steady-state activity such as long-distance running in which a high cardiorespiratory efficiency is essential. The cross-country runners were similar in physique to those middle- and long-distance runners measured by *Hay and Watson* [1970] and those measured by *Malina* et al. [1971]. This latter study also obtained similar anthropometric data and percent fat in their distance runners. *Pipes* [1977] and *Wilmore and Brown* [1974] reported even higher densities and lower percent fat in their women distance runners.

The physiques of the basketball players were similar to those of the Canadian basketball players measured by *Alexander* [1976] in height, weight, ponderal index and somatotype. Though of similar height they are lighter and more ectomorphic than the elite women basketball players measured by *Vaccaro* et al. [1979]. They had slightly higher percent fat than *Vaccaro's* group and those women basketball players measured by *Sinning* [1973]. The tallness of the basketball players in this investigation suggests that height is an important factor to success in basketball. *Alexander* [1976] concluded that: 'Height of female basketball players is a good predictor of basketball performance, rebounding ability and points scored'. As in a similar study of 14 groups of top sportsmen [*Maas*, 1974], the women basketball players were both tallest and heaviest.

There was considerable variation in somatotype and in percent fat in the groups of modern educational gymnasts and swimmers. However, their mean somatotypes were very similar and both fell in the central area of the somatochart. Like other physical education students [*Bale*, 1978, 1979, 1980; *Carter*, 1965; *Cockerham*, 1975] they were generally less fat and more muscular than non-physical education students. The gymnasts were more endomorphic and had higher percent fat than those gymnasts measured by *Falls and Humphrey* [1978] and they were heavier and fatter than the Springfield College women gymnastics team measured by *Sinning and Lindberg* [1972]. It should be noted, however, that the philosophy of modern educational gymnastics is to suit the activity to the physique rather than select a particular physique most suitable for the activity as in more formal and Olympic gymnastics.

The swimmers had similar percent fat to those reported by *Katch and McArdle* [1973]. The few that performed in the sprint swimming events

Somatotype of Sportswomen

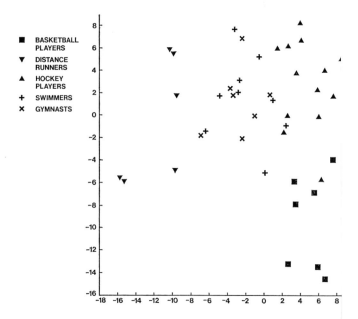

Fig. 2. Five different groups of sportswomen using the first two canon

Table IV. The first two canonical variables evaluated at group means

Sports group	1st canonical variable	2nd cano
Hockey players	5.47	3.02
Cross-country runners	−13.01	−2.02
Basketball players	5.06	−9.30
Swimming team	−2.31	2.44
Gymnastics team	−2.67	1.40

The canonical variables were formed from the original 19 standardised vari

The hockey girls were slightly heavier, though similar in hei; girls of their age. Their somatotypes indicate that they too are mo and less fat than non-athletic girls. They are also less endomorpl New Zealand women hockey players measured by *Johnston ɛ* [1968]. The New Zealand girls were also shorter and lighter tha lish hockey players.

were more muscular and less fat than the rest of the group. No relationship was found between physique and type of swimming stroke in this small sample of swimmers measured.

As can be seen from tables II and III, the ballet dancers are lightest. They had similar heights and ponderal indices to those of the cross-country runners and they were the lightest of all the groups. It must be remembered, however, that they were younger and a few of the girls, therefore, may not have completed their adolescent development. The lean body weight of the dancers was the lowest, yet they had a higher percent fat than the cross-country runners and athletes. All the ballet dancers were full-time members of the Royal Ballet School. As they do approximately 6–7 h ballet training each day in addition to their performances, one would have expected a higher lean body weight to fat ratio. Perhaps nutrition and dieting are important factors here.

The women athletes consisted of 6 sprinters, 2 pentathletes and 3 throwers (discus and javelin), of international standard. As a group, they were similar in physique to the track-and-field athletes of *Malina* et al. [1971] and those measured by *Brown and Wilmore* [1971]. The 6 sprinters had less fat and were shorter and lighter than the pentathletes and throwers. The mean heights and weights of the sprinters were 164.8 cm and 56.1 kg compared with 172.8 cm and 64.3 kg for the pentathletes and 172.6 cm and 66.8 kg for the throwers. The athletes were also taller, heavier and had more fat and lean body weight than the cross-country runners. These findings also agree with those of *Malina* et al. [1971], *Hay and Watson* [1970] and *Pipes* [1977]. It would seem, therefore, that physique and body composition, to a large degree, dictate a person's success in track-and-field events.

The cyclists competed in a wide range of events at national level including sprint, pursuit and road races. As for the athletes, there was a wide distribution of height, weight and body composition within the group. The sprint and pursuit cyclists were heavier both in fat and lean body weight than the road racers.

To summarise, it appears that sportswomen are generally more muscular and less fat than non-athletic women and as such are more successful in sport. It is difficult to separate training, greater participation in physical activity and genetic factors from the physical parameters described, all of which contribute to a successful performance. However, it is suggested that success is due in part to the significant positive relationship of mesomorphy to physical performance. If one accepts that there is some validity in the relationship of temperament with physique [*Sheldon* et al., 1940] the temperament associated with mesomorphy of a more aggressive, assertive and competitive personality is also most related to success in sport.

Summary

This paper examines the discriminative power of measurements of physique between female competitors in different sports. Physique and body composition was assessed from anthropometric measurements. A canonical analysis separated the sportswomen into distinct groups on the basis of a combination of weight, height, percent fat, femur bone width, and biceps girth. Hockey and basketball players scored high on these variables in contrast to cross-country runners, who had similar physiques to the ballet dancers. The dancers had the lowest percent fats, were smallest and lightest. The hockey players, gymnasts and swimmers had balanced physiques. The basketball players were significantly taller than the other sports groups. The findings of this study suggest that sportswomen are more muscular and less fat than non-athletic women and their success in sport is due in part to the relationship of this muscle to physical performance.

References

Alexander, M.J.L.: The relationship of somatotype and selected anthropometric measures of basketball performance in highly skilled females. Res. Quart. 47: 575–585 (1976).

Bale, P.: The physiques of physical education students and their relationships to performance. Res. Papers phys. Ed. 3: 30–33 (1978).

Bale, P.: The relationship between physique and basic motor performance in a group of female physical education students. Res. Papers phys. Ed. 1: 26–32 (1979).

Bale, P.: The relationship of physique and body composition to strength in a group of P.E. students. Br. J. Sports Med. December (1980).

Behnke, A.R.; Wilmore, J.H.: Evaluation and regulation of body build and composition (Prentice Hall, Englewood Cliffs 1974).

Brown, W.J.; Jones, P.R.: The distribution of body fat in relation to habitual activity. Ann. hum. Biol. 4: 537–550 (1977).

Brown, C.H.; Wilmore, J.H.: Physical and physiological profiles of champion women long-distance runners. Med. Sci. Sports 3 (1971).

Carter, J.E.L.: The physiques of female physical education teachers in training. Phys. Ed. 57: 6–16 (1965).

Carter, J.E.L.: The somatotype of athletes – a review. Hum. Biol. 42: 535–569 (1970).

Cockerham, B.W.: Physiques of arts and physical education students. N.Z. J. Hlth PE Recr. 8: 62–66 (1975).

Durnin, J.V.; Rahaman, M.M.: The assessment of the amount of fat in the human body from measurements of skinfold thickness. Br. J. Nutr. 21: 681–689 (1967).

Durnin, J.V.; Womersley, J.: Body fat assessed from total body density and its estimation from skinfold thickness measurements on 481 men and women aged from 16–72 years. Br. J. Nutr. 32: 77–97 (1974).

Falls, H.B.; Humphrey, L.D.: Body type and composition differences between placers and nonplacers in AIAW gymnastics Meet. Res. Quart. *49:* 38–43 (1978).

Garay, A.L. de; Levine, L.; Carter, J.E.L.: Genetic and anthropological studies of Olympic athletes (Academic Press, London 1974).

Gayton, P.H.: The physique of New Zealand surf life savers. N.Z. J. Hlth PE Recr. *8:* 114–120 (1975).

Hay, J.C.; Watson, J.M.: The somatotypes of women track and field athletes. N.Z. J. Hlth PE Recr. *3:* 28–49 (1970).

Hirata, K.: Physique and age of Tokyo Olympic champions. J. Sports Med. phys. Fit. *6:* 207–222 (1966).

Johnston, R.E.; Watson, J.M.: A comparison of the phenotypes of women basketball and hockey players. N.Z. J. Hlth PE Recr. *40:* 48–54 (1968).

Katch, F.; McArdle, W.: Prediction of body density from simple anthropometric measurements. Hum. Biol. *45:* 445–454 (1973).

Leek, G.M.: The physique of swimming champions. N.Z. J. Hlth PE Recr. *2:* 30–41 (1969).

Lewis, A.S.: The physique of New Zealand basketball players. N.Z. J. PE *39:* 25–36 (1966).

Mass, G.D.: The physique of athletes (Leiden University Press, Leiden 1974).

Malina, R.M.; Harper, A.B.; Avent, H.A.; Campbell, D.E.: Physique of female track and field athletes. Med. Sci. Sports *3:* 32–38 (1971).

Maxwell, A.E.: Multivariate analysis; some problems in the discrimination and classification of psychiatric patients. 5th Int. Science Meet. of the Int. Epidemiological Ass. (Institute of Psychiatry, London 1968).

Parnell, R.W.: Behaviour and physique (Arnold, London 1958).

Pipes, T.V.: Body composition characteristics of male and female track and field athletes. Res. Quart. *48:* 244–247 (1977).

Sheldon, W.H.; Dupertuis, C.W.; McDermott, E.: Atlas of men (Harper, New York 1954).

Sheldon, W.H.; Stevens, S.S.; Tucker, W.B.: The varieties of human physiques (Harper, New York 1940).

Sinning, W.E.: Body composition, cardiorespiratory function and rule changes in women's basketball. Res. Quart. *44:* 313–321 (1973).

Sinning, W.E.; Cunningham, L.N.; Racaniello, A.P.; Sholes, J.L.: Body composition and somatotype of male and female Nordic skiers. Res. Quart. *49:* 741–749 (1978).

Sinning, W.E.; Lindberg, G.D.: Physical characteristics of college age women gymnasts. Res. Quart. *43:* 226–234 (1972).

Siri, W.E.: The gross composition of the body; in Lawrence, Tobias, Advances in biological and medical physics, vol. 4, pp. 239–280 (Academic Press, New York 1956).

Tanner, J.M.: The physique of the Olympic athlete (Allen & Unwin, London 1964).

Tatsuoka, M.: Multivariate analysis (Wiley, New York 1971).

Vaccaro, P.; Clarke, D.H.; Wrenn, J.P.: Physiological profiles of élite women basketball players. J. Sports Med. *19:* 45–54 (1979).

Wilmore, J.H.; Brown, C.H.: Physiological profiles of women distance runners. Med. Sci. Sports *6:* 178–181 (1974).

Dr. P. Bale, Chelsea School of Human Movement, Brighton Polytechnic, Milnthorpe Court, 57 Meads Road, Eastbourne BN20 7AD (England)

Medicine Sport, vol. 15, pp. 168–175 (Karger, Basel 1981)

Differences in Males and Females in Joint Movement Range during Growth

F. Merni, M. Balboni, S. Bargellini, G. Menegatti

Departments of Topographical Anatomy, Bologna University, Italy; Human Anatomy Applied to Physical Education, Bologna ISEF, Italy

Introduction

The ability to move or flex a joint throughout a complete range is of fundamental importance in physical education and sport, permitting optimum utilization of strength and speed, and facilitating the learning and coordination of motor skills.

Many studies of joint mobility have been done, but the results appear contradictory. Studies indicating least flexibility between the ages of 10 and 12 years [*Phillips* et al., 1955; *Kirchner and Glines*, 1957; *Buxton*, 1957], and greatest flexibility between 15 and 16 years [*Zaciorskij*, 1974], seem to be confirmed by the toe-touch test of *Fleishman* [1964] and *Sykora* [1967]; yet *Clarke* [1975] and *Krahenbuhl and Martin* [1977] report a decrease in joint mobility from 10 to 12 onwards. It is reported by some of the above authors that girls are more flexible than boys throughout the growth period, and *de Vries* [1971] considers that the situation continues throughout adult life.

The aim of the study, therefore, was to investigate differences in joint movement range with regard to sex and age, using easily administered tests, which would readily identify joint flexibility. This would both permit the establishment of norms for individual comparison and enable teachers to select movement requirements appropriate to age and sex abilities. In addition, it was hoped to elucidate the findings of previous studies in this area.

Methods

Static flexibility is usually measured directly at the joint (with a goniometer) or indirectly (with linear measurements), by the position of the body parts forming one or both the angle arms. There are no tests available which will give an overall assessment of joint range movement due to the specificity of joint movement [*Harris*, 1969; *Derzsy*, 1973; *Bargellini*, 1979], but identification of the hip, shoulder and trunk joints as being the most important in terms of sports performances [*Vaszil'ev*, 1963] led to these being chosen for this study.

Subjects

460 boys and 360 girls, aged 6–18 from several Bologna schools were divided into groups according to sex and age (with age group intervals of 1 year), and measured at some period between 8 a.m. and 8 p.m. Each group was divided into subgroups on the basis of height and subgroups were tested at random during the group test period.

Instruments

The following instruments were used: A goniometer attached to a height-adjustable (1 m²) board and calibrated in 5° units, adapted from *Correnti* [1974] and *Merni* [1977]. Goniometric compasses calibrated in 2° units. A 50-cm board (calibrated in centimetres), fixed on a 32-cm high box. A 120-cm long stick, of 2.5 cm diameter, graduated in 5-cm units.

Procedures

Extension and flexion of both hips and trunk were measured using the board goniometer, by two testers – one controlling the fixed body part (upper or lower), and the other measuring the angle achieved at the limit of movement by moving the body part.

The centre of the goniometer was positioned at the greater trochanter and the position of the 7th cervical vertebral apophysis was used to indicate trunk flexion/extension with the legs straight and maintained in a vertical position throughout. With the trunk fixed vertically, the position of the head of the fibula was used to indicate hip flexion/extension; in hip flexion the knee of the engaged leg was flexed, while in hip extension the leg was straight. Abduction of the hips was measured in a sitting position with the back vertically supported against a wall and the legs extended. The angle between the abducted thighs was measured with a goniometric compass. The 'sit and reach' test [*Wells and Dillon*, 1952; *Gombos*, 1974] was performed in the long sitting position with the subject sliding his hands forward on the 50-cm board, measurement being taken at the limit of fingertip reach. Shoulder mobility was measured with the 120 cm stick, the subject being required to rotate the arms about a transverse axis whilst gripping the stick with both hands. The narrowest grip that the subject could maintain without flexion of arms or trunk during a backward/forward rotation was measured. All measurements were preceded by a standard warm-up with particular attention being paid to the chosen joints. As to the reliability of such movements, we noticed coefficients between 0.79 and 0.97 for symmetrical tests on reduced samples. Values were smaller for hip flexion and extension, especially in younger children (about 0.60), maybe because of the difficulty in understanding the movement and the lack of coordination.

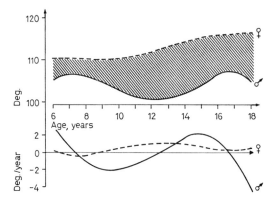

Fig. 1. Flexibility of trunk (forward flexion) in girls and boys, 6–18 years.

Statistical Evaluation

The collected linear and angular data were analysed on the CDC 6600 Computer of North-East Italy Interuniversity Computer Centre. A 5th degree polynomial was fitted for each test through individual points by the least-squares method. Values of mobility as a function of age (measured in months) were plotted as the trend of the computed derivative so as to highlight curve maxima/minima and slope features. A 5th degree polynomial was chosen in order to permit a satisfactory trend description through the computed derivative. The Student's t-test was used to identify significant differences in mobility due to age and sex.

Results

Diagonal shading in the figures indicate the existence of a significant difference between the two sexes ($p < 0.05$). The bottom part of each figure shows the result of fitting a 5th degree polynomial to the data to indicate velocity changes in flexibility with age. However, caution should be exercised in the interpretation of such curves since the data are cross-sectional and not longitudinal.

Trunk Flexion. Both girls and boys displayed a decrease in trunk flexibility before puberty (minimum at 9 for girls and 12 for boys) followed by a gradual increase until the ages of 16–18, either measurements were in degrees or in cm in the 'sit and reach test'. The loss of flexibility was greater amongst boys (fig. 1) with the result that the subsequent increase only returned them to their former level. The girls, however, improved their flexi-

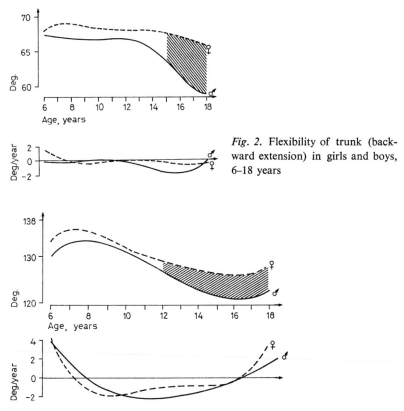

Fig. 2. Flexibility of trunk (backward extension) in girls and boys, 6–18 years

Fig. 3. Flexibility of right hip (flexion) in girls and boys, 6–18 years.

bility beyond their initial level prior to decrease. At all times, girls displayed a greater trunk flexibility than boys.

Trunk Extension. Trunk extensibility reduced in both sexes with increasing age. A significant difference was identified between the two sexes at the post elementary school level (fig. 2).

Hip Flexion. The results (fig. 3) were similar to those for trunk extension, indicating a progressive decrease with age to a minimum at 16–18 years. A feature of this test was that the difference between the two sexes was greater for right hip flexion than for left. It should be noted that this one was the only test in which differences between successive age groups (from 9 to 12) were significant ($p < 0.05$).

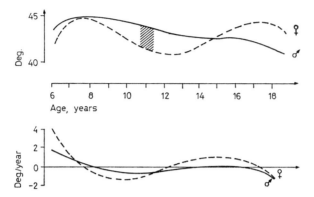

Fig. 4. Flexibility of right hip (extension) in girls and boys, 6–18 years.

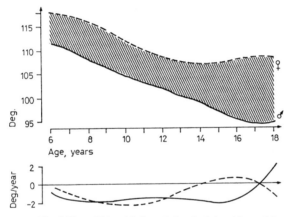

Fig. 5. Flexibility of hips (sitting abduction) in girls and boys, 6–18 years.

Hip Extension. Boys exhibited a general decrease in extensibility with age, but girls showed a quite different pattern to those found in the other tests (fig. 4). They demonstrated a decrease to a minimum at 12–13 and then an increase to the original level. This middle years decrease highlighted the only case in which boys had a greater range of movement than girls, though the difference was only significant for a short period around the age of 11.

Abduction. At first a continuous decline with age was shown by both sexes (fig. 5) with significant differences seen between the two sexes; then

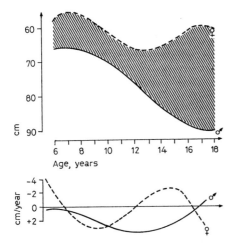

Fig. 6. Flexibility of shoulder (sagittal stick rotation).

differences become more and more significant because, while males show a further decline, females reach a steady state.

Shoulder Rotation. A pattern, similar to that found during hip extension tests, was found in this test with the continuing decrease in male flexibility opposed by an increase in females from the ages of 12–16 (fig. 6), with resultant extreme differences at 16–18 very clearly indicated.

Discussion

The results clearly show greater joint mobility in females. The reasons for this are not clear-cut. There are a number of factors which could influence range of movement, e.g. structure of bone and cartilage; action of joint capsules, fascial sheaths, ligaments and tendons; strength of agonist muscles, and the stretching capacities of antagonist muscles, tendons and ligaments; yet these influences vary for every joint and for every movement.

It is well established that agonist muscle strength increase with age, yet greater strength capacity does not seem to effect range of movement. In a previous work [*Merni* et al., 1979] the correlation between static or explosive strength tests and movement range tests were negative and low.

The decrease in mobility with age support similar findings by *Clarke* [1975] and *Krahenbuhl and Martin* [1977]. In general, the loss of flexibility is greater for boys, while there is an apparent post-pubertal improvement in girls. The activity of the female sex hormones on the stretch capacities of muscle and connective tissue may provide a basis for this improvement since softening of connective tissues, and hence greater joint movement, at the sacroiliac and symphysis pubis joints are concomitants of pregnancy. Boys, however, also demonstrate a post-pubertal increase in one of the tests, i.e. forward trunk flexion. In this particular test, the ages of minimum flexion – 9–10 for girls and 12 for boys – coincided with those identified by *Phillips* et al. [1955], *Kirchner and Glines* [1957] and *Buxton* [1957]. It is thought that the subsequent improvement in mobility is a result of an increasing advantage of those factors aiding movement, e.g. abdominal strength, over those factors limiting it (among the most important of which, according to *Fieldman* [1968], is the extensibility of the hamstring muscles).

We conclude that mobility is joint-specific and thus different joints cannot be adequately compared, a point which may explain apparent disagreement between authors in previous studies. Whereas we can readily identify trends in flexibility at specific joints, we cannot draw general conclusions about joint mobility throughout the whole body, nor identify specific causative factors for either increases or decreases in flexibility.

Summary

460 boys and 360 girls from 6 to 18 years were measured for range of trunk, hip and shoulder movement. Curves were fitted using a 5th degree polynomial, and a Student's t-test used to test for significant differences in range due to sex and age. In general, the ranges for females were found to be greater than those for males. Male values tended to decrease with age (with one exception), whereas in some of the tests girls displayed an opposing trend.

References

Bargellini, S.: Rapporti esistenti tra la mobilità di alcune articolazioni nell'età evolutiva; Tesi diploma ISEF (Bologna 1979).
Buxton, D.: Extension of the Kraus-Weber test. Res. Quart. *28:* 210–217 (1957).
Clarke, H.H.: Joint and body range of movement. Phys. Fit. Res. Dig. *5:* 16–18 (1975).
Correnti, V.: Instrument and technique to measure trunk flexibility; in Schönholzer, Standardization of physical fitness test, p. 71 (Birkhäuser, Basel 1974).

Derzsy, B.: Probàk és elemzések az izületi mozgékonysag vizsgàlatàban. Tudom. Közlem. *III/IV:* 63–81 (1973).

Fieldman, H.: Relative contribution of the back and hamstring muscles in the performance of the toe-touch test after selected extensibility exercises. Res. Quart. *39:* 518–523 (1968).

Fleishman, E.A.: The structure and measurement of physical fitness, pp. 121–126 (Prentice-Hall, Englewood Cliffs 1964).

Gombos, M.: Probàk az edzettség mérésére, pp. 82–89 (Magyar Testnevelési Föiskola, Budapest 1974).

Harris, M.L.: A factor analytic study of flexibility. Res. Quart. *40:* 62–70 (1969).

Kirchner, G.; Glines, D.: Comparative analysis of Eugene, Oregon, elementary school children using the Kraus-Weber test of minimum muscular fitness. Res. Quart. *28:* 16–25 (1957).

Krahenbuhl, G.S.; Martin, S.L.: Adolescent body size and flexibility. Res. Quart. *48:* 797–799 (1977).

Merni, F.; Dala, D.; Grandi, E.; Facondini, G.; Capizzi, C.: Relazioni tra le capacità motorie e loro sviluppo nei ragazzi di un centro di avviamento all'atletica. Atletica-studi 10–12, pp. 173–198 (1979).

Merni, S.: Mobilità sagittale e trasversale del busto e delle articolazioni della spalla e dell'anca e sue variazioni durante il 1° semestre di frequenza all'ISEF; Tesi di diploma ISEF, Roma (1977).

Phillips, M. et al.: Analysis of results from the Kraus-Weber test of minimum muscular fitness in children. Res. Quart. *26:* 314–323 (1955).

Sykora, F.: L'éducation physique dans la formation attitudinaire chez les jeunes agés entre 7 et 15 ans de la ville de Bratislava; in Atti congresso europeo di educazione fisica, pp. 285–303 (Centro studi per l'educazione fisica, Bologna 1967).

Vaszil'ev, E.P.: Kak kontrolirovat razvitie gibkoszti u skolnikov. Fizics. Kul. V Skole *4:* 12–16 (1963).

Vries, H.A. de: Physiology of exercise; 3rd ed., pp. 360–370 (Staples Press, London 1971).

Wells, K.F.; Dillon, E.K.: Sit and reach, a test of back and leg flexibility. Res. Quart. *23:* 115–118 (1952).

Zaciorskij, V.M.: Le qualità fisiche dello sportivo; 1st ed., p. 170 (Ed. Atletica Leggera, Milano 1974).

Dr. F. Merni, Cattedra di Anatomia Topografica,
Via Irnerio 48, I-40126 Bologna (Italy)

Medicine Sport, vol. 15, pp. 176–185 (Karger, Basel 1981)

Somatic and Motor Characteristics of Female Gymnasts

G. Beunen, A. Claessens, M. van Esser

Kinanthropometric Research Unit, Institute of Physical Education, K.U. Leuven, Leuven, Belgium

Introduction

Since *Kohlrausch's* [1929] report concerning the physique of Olympic athletes numerous studies have been published describing the somatic characteristics of outstanding athletes competing in various sports disciplines.

Mostly due to the unique contributions of *Tanner* [1964], *Tittel* [1968], *Carter* [1970], *Tittel and Wutscherk* [1972], *Eiben* [1972], *Stepnicka* [1972], *de Garay* et al. [1974], *Maas* [1974], and *Jungman* [1976] more insight has been gained into the body build, body composition, and somatotype of athletes.

In discussing these studies *Carter* [1978] concluded that: '... in terms of absolute somatotype, absolute and relative body dimensions, and body composition clear prototypes exist for outstanding performances requiring strength, speed and stamina.' Moreover, in reviewing the physiological characteristics of male and female athletes, *Wilmore* [1979] found that male and female athletes are similar in lower body strength (expressed per unit of body weight), cardiovascular endurance capacity, body composition, and muscle fiber type. He stated further that: 'What once appeared to be dramatic biological differences in physiological function between the sexes, may, in fact, be more related to cultural and social restrictions placed on the female as she attains puberty, i.e. a sedentary life style.'

However, little has been published about the motor abilities of outstanding athletes. From a kinanthropometric viewpoint, it seems therefore of interest to gather more information about these motor abilities together with the physiological and anthropometric characteristics. Therefore, the aim of this study was to investigate the somatic and motor profiles of Belgian female gymnasts and to compare their results with those of a reference population and outstanding female gymnasts from other populations.

Materials and Methods

Data were collected from a sample of 23 female gymnasts from the three 'federations' of Belgium. 18 girls were members of the national team and 5 girls, 1 of 11 years and 4 of 14 years, although not yet selected for the team, already regularly attended the national training sessions. In addition to a large number (39) of anthropometric measurements, a motor ability test battery [*Simons* et al., 1969] was administered. Several other parameters were investigated: cardiorespiratory parameters, age at menarche, skeletal age determined from an X-ray of the left hand and wrist, three standardized photographs for the estimation of the somatotype. Other factors such as sociocultural background of their families, sports participation, family composition, training, preferred discipline, and results in gymnastic competition were researched by means of an interview and questionnaire.

Skeletal age was determined according to the Tanner-Whitehouse II method [*Tanner* et al., 1975] and the anthropometric somatotype was estimated according to Heath-Carter [*Carter*, 1975]. All measurements, codifications and ratings were done by trained kin-anthropometrists. An overview of the different measurements is given in table I. As a reference population, a sample of 450 girls was taken from one school in Leuven. The body dimensions, the maturity status, and the somatotype components were also compared with the results of other samples of female gymnasts as reported in literature.

Results

Comparison with a Reference Population

The chronological age of the gymnasts ranged from 11.4 years to 21.4 years with a mean value of 16.6 years. The individual values of the body measurements were plotted on the z-score profiles of the reference samples of the same age level (table II). Gymnasts have smaller body dimensions than the reference group except for biacromial width and upper arm circumference. Relative to their height, they are short in the trunk and have a relative large muscle mass. Gymnasts are also small in the hips relative to their biacromial width.

The mean somatotype of the gymnasts was 2.4–3.7–3.1. The mean age at menarche for 13 of the 23 girls studied was $15.13 \pm SD$ 1.70 years. The mean chronological age of the girls who did not yet reach this milestone was 14.4 years. However, the mean age at menarche for Belgian samples

Table I. Measurements and tests administered to 23 female gymnasts

Anthropometry	*Motor ability test battery*
Weight	Flamingo balance (balance)
Height	Stick balance (eye-hand coordination)
Sitting height	Plate tapping
Leg length	Sit and reach (flexibility)
Total arm length	Vertical jump (explosive strength)
Forearm length	Arm pull (static strength)
Tibia length	Leg lifts (trunk strength)
Biacromial diameter	Bent arm hang (functional strength)
Chest width	Shuttle run (running speed)
Biiliac diameter	Handgrip (R & L)
Biepicondylar femur (R & L)	
Biepicondylar humerus (R & L)	*Cardiorespiratory parameters*
Upper arm flexed (R & L)	Pulse frequency at rest and after exercise
Thigh circumference (R & L)	Forced vital capacity
Calf circumference (R & L)	Blood pressure at rest and after exercise
Chest circumference	Forced expired volume
Subscapular skinfold (R & L)	Peak flow
Suprailiac skinfold (R & L)	
Triceps skinfold (R & L)	*Maturity indicators*
Calf skinfold (R & L)	Age at menarche
Biceps skinfold[a]	Skeletal age (TWII)
Cheek skinfold[a]	
Chin skinfold[a]	*Somatotype (Heath-Carter)*
Chest 1 skinfold[a]	*Sociocultural inquiry*
Chest 2 skinfold[a]	Gymnastic results
Abdominal skinfold[a]	Training
Thigh skinfold[a]	Sports practice
Percentage fat[b]	Family composition, sociocultural
Density[b]	determinants

R & L = Measured on both sides; a according to *Parizkova* [1977]; b according to *Durnin and Rahaman* [1967].

studied recently varied between 12.8 and 13.0 years [*Jeurissen*, 1969; *Beunen* et al., 1978], which indicates that female gymnasts were markedly retarded relative to the Belgian population. Their skeletal development was also retarded. For 11 girls whose chronological age varied between 16.1 and 21.4 years, an adult skeletal maturity was found (TW2 technique). For the remaining 11 girls (for 1 girl the X-ray was missing), a mean difference of 1.5 years was found between their chronological and skeletal ages. With

Table II. Frequency distribution of the individual body dimensions of female gymnasts plotted within the age category of each gymnast

Body dimension	Individual value ≤ −1SD	−1SD < indiv. value < +1SD	Individual value ≥ +1SD
Weight	12	10	1
Height	11	5	4
Sitting height	12	11	0
Leg length	4	14	5
Biacromial diameter	2	13	8
Biiliac diameter	16	7	2
Biepicondylar humerus	10	13	0
Biepicondylar femur	12	11	0
Upper arm flexed	3	17	3
Thigh circumference	10	12	1
Calf circumference	7	13	1
Triceps skinfold	13	10	0
Biceps skinfold	10	13	0
Subscapular skinfold	16	7	0
Suprailiac skinfold	11	12	0

Table III. Frequency distribution of the individual motor abilities plotted within the age category of each gymnast (n = 23)

Test	Individual value ≤ −1SD	−1SD < indiv. value < +1SD	Individual value ≥ +1SD
Vertical jump	1	4	18
Sit and reach	0	0	23
Leg lifts	0	1	22
Plate tapping	1	16	6
Arm pull	0	4	19
Bent arm hang	0	10	13

the exception of 1 girl (chronological age equals 11.4 years), none of the girls studied was advanced in skeletal development, and for 3 of them a difference of 2.5–3.0 years was observed between their chronological and skeletal ages.

We compared the motor performance of the gymnasts with samples of comparable age levels (table III). Female gymnasts earned extremely high scores in flexibility (sit and reach) and in trunk strength (leg lifts). Their

Table IV. Comparison of somatic characteristics of female gymnasts from four different samples

Somatic characteristics	Author			
	Sinning and Lindberg [1972] (n=14)	Zaharieva et al. [1979] (n=106)	de Garay et al. [1974] (n=21)	Belgian sample (n=23)
Height, cm	158.1 ± 5.04	158.6 ± 5.39	156.9 ± 5.1	158.4 ± 9.21
Weight, kg	51.1 ± 7.08	50.7 ± 6.47	49.8 ± 4.5	49.6 ± 9.69
Sitting height, cm	–	84.2 ± 3.06	–	82.1 ± 4.01
Leg length, cm	–	74.4 ± 4.18	–	76.3 ± 6.03
Biacromial diameter, cm	35.1 ± 1.95	35.4 ± 1.95	35.7 ± 1.7	35.3 ± 2.36
Biiliac diameter, cm	25.7 ± 1.23	25.8 ± 1.39	25.6 ± 1.3	24.6 ± 1.85
Biepicondylar humerus L, cm	5.7 ± 0.23	–	–	5.7 ± 0.38
Biepicondylar humerus R, cm	5.7 ± 0.27	–	–	5.8 ± 0.38
Biepicondylar femur L, cm	8.5 ± 0.29	–	–	8.1 ± 0.38
Biepicondylar femur R, cm	8.4 ± 0.31	–	–	8.2 ± 0.36
Chest circumference inspiration, cm	–	83.2 ± 5.09	–	87.0 ± 7.10
Chest circumference expiration, cm	–	77.1 ± 4.79	–	80.4 ± 6.53
Upper arm flexed L, cm	26.4 ± 2.05	26.3 ± 1.92	–	26.6 ± 2.75
Upper arm flexed R, cm	–	26.6 ± 4.50	–	26.7 ± 2.63
Thigh circumference L, cm	51.4 ± 4.09	49.9 ± 3.11	–	51.1 ± 4.78
Thigh circumference R, cm	–	50.2 ± 3.07	–	51.2 ± 4.91
Calf circumference L, cm	33.4 ± 1.52	33.6 ± 2.21	–	32.5 ± 2.64
Calf circumference R, cm	–	33.7 ± 2.22	–	32.6 ± 2.75
Handgrip L, kg	–	31.9 ± 6.11	–	32.6 ± 7.88
Handgrip R, kg	–	34.1 ± 5.76	–	34.6 ± 9.51

results in explosive strength (vertical jump), static strength (arm pull), and functional strength (bent arm hang) were also above average. However, only an average result was obtained for speed of limb movement (plate tapping). In all of the cases the results for flexibility (sit and reach) were above $\overline{X} + 1$ SD and for speed of limb movement 16 out of 23 girls obtained results between $\overline{X} \pm 1$ SD.

Comparison with Other Samples of Female Gymnasts

Table IV shows that there are striking similarities in the mean absolute body dimensions of the four samples under consideration. It should be men-

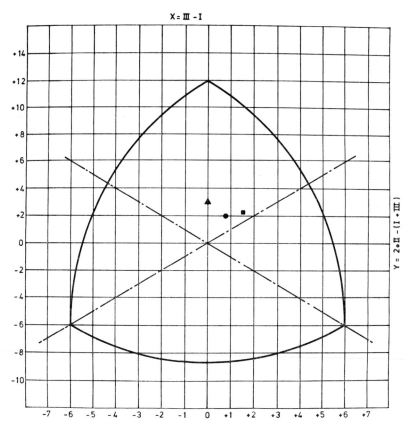

Fig. 1. Mean somatotypes of female gymnasts from three samples ▲=Olympic [gymnasts, Mexico [*de Garay* et al., 1974]; ■=International Championship, Cuba 1977 *Lopez* et al., 1979]; ●=Belgian gymnasts (present study).

tioned that the gymnasts studied by *Zaharieva* et al. [1979] and by *de Garay* et al. [1974] were outstanding athletes, which is not necessarily the case for the sample of college women studied by *Sinning and Lindberg* [1972]. However, it is noteworthy that for the Belgian sample larger standard deviations are found for nearly all somatic characteristics. This larger variability is mainly due to the greater age range studied and especially due to the inclusion of the results of one 11.4-year-old girl.

As shown in figure 1, the mean somatotype of Belgian gymnasts was situated between the mean somatotype of Olympic gymnasts in Mexico [*de Garay* et al., 1974] (mean somatotype equals 2.7–4.2–2.8), and the par-

Table V. Age at menarche in three different samples of female gymnasts

Author(s)	n	Age at menarche	
		mean	SD
Malina et al. [1979] Montreal Olympiad	11	14.50	0.82
Märker [1979] GDR gymnasts	25	15.04	1.06
Present study Belgian gymnasts	13	15.13	1.70

ticipants of an International Championship in Cuba in 1977 [*Lopez* et al., 1979] (mean somatotype equals 2.0–3.9–3.5). The Belgians (mean somatotype equals 2.4–3.7–3.1) obtained somewhat lower values in endomorphy and mesomorphy and higher values in ectomorphy than did the Olympic competitors.

The mean age at menarche observed in this study is in close agreement with the age reported by *Märker* [1979] for GDR gymnasts. However, the mean age for the Belgians is older than the age found for competitors in the Montreal Olympics (table V) [*Malina*, 1980]. As for sexual development, an average delay of 1.5 years was found for skeletal development which confirms the findings of *Novotny and Taftlova* [1971] obtained with so-called 'Olympic hopes'.

Conclusions

The female gymnasts studied herein have small body dimensions when compared to reference populations of the same age and sex. They are small in the hips and broad in the shoulders and have a relatively short trunk. They obtain high results in several motor tests, especially in flexibility and trunk strength, and above average scores in static, functional and explosive strength. Belgian gymnasts are also delayed in sexual and skeletal maturity.

These good performances and delayed maturation seem rather contradictory but, as was suggested by *Malina* [1980], it could perhaps be explained by the following two-part hypothesis: (1) At the extreme of the performance continuum better performers were more commonly later maturing and linear in physique [*Beunen* et al., 1978]. Therefore, the physique characteristics of late-maturing girls are perhaps more suitable for successful athletic performance. (2) With the attainment of menarche the early-maturing girl is perhaps socialized away from athletic competition through a myriad of social and status-related motives. Since the late-maturing girls are older chronologically when they reach age at menarche and are also different in physique, they have perhaps not experienced the social pressures regarding competitive sports for girls and/or are more able to cope with these pressures [*Malina*, 1980, pp. 43, 44].

The mean somatotype of the Belgian female gymnasts is also in fairly good agreement with the mean somatotype of gymnasts who compete in international championships. Mainly due to the inclusion of a young girl in the sample studied a larger variability in anthropometric measurements was found in comparison with other samples reported in the literature. However, striking similarities were found in the average somatic characteristics, although the samples under consideration were from different populations studied during the last decade. During this decade there could have been an increase in the body dimensions of the populations. In a recent overview on secular trend *Roche* [1979] concluded that: 'In summary, evidence accumulates that the secular trend is slowing down or has ceased for many middle and upper socioeconomic groups in developed countries.' In our opinion it seems likely that the similarities reported here reflect perhaps a better 'sampling' by gymnast talent scouts or trainers.

Considering the very high scores in motor abilities, the characteristic sexual and skeletal retardation, the similarities in the average somatotype components and body measurements between the Belgian sample and other samples of female gymnasts, we rather believe that the fairly poor performance of the Belgians in the international competitions is affected by other factors rather than somatic or motor characteristics.

Summary

This study was designed to investigate the somatic and motor profiles of Belgian female gymnasts and to compare their results with those of a reference population and those of other outstanding gymnasts.

A large number of somatic, motor, and cardiorespiratory parameters were examined in 23 female gymnasts together with their competition results and their sociocultural background. This research showed that female gymnasts have small body dimensions, are of a more masculine build, and are more mesomorphic and less endomorphic and ectomorphic than a reference population. These results have been reinforced in other studies of outstanding female gymnasts. Belgian gymnasts have very good flexibility and trunk strength and are above average for static, explosive, and functional strength. Female gymnasts are also markedly retarded in biological maturity.

Considering these results it was concluded that the fairly poor results of the Belgian female gymnasts during international competitions seem to be affected by other factors rather than simply somatic or motor characteristics.

References

Beunen, G.; Beul, G. de; Ostyn, M.; Renson, R.; Simons, J.; Gerven, D. van: Age of menarche and motor performance in girls aged 11 through 18; in Borms, Hebbelinck, Pediatric work physiology. Medicine Sport, vol. 11, pp. 118–123 (Karger, Basel 1978).

Carter, J.E.L.: The somatotype of athletes – a review. Hum. Biol. *42:* 535–569 (1970).

Carter, J.E.L.: The Heath-Carter somatotype method (San Diego State University, San Diego 1975).

Carter, J.E.L.: Prediction of outstanding athletic ability: the structural perspective; in Landry, Orban, Exercise physiology, vol. IV, pp. 29–42 (Symposia Specialists, Miami 1978).

Durnin, J.V.G.A.; Rahaman, M.M.: The assessment of the amounts of fat in the human body from measurements of skinfold thickness. Br. J. Nutr. *21:* 681–689 (1967).

Eiben, O.: The physique of women athletes (The Hungarian Scientific Council for Physical Education, Budapest 1972).

Garay, A.L. de; Levine, L.; Carter, J.E.L.: Genetic and anthropological studies of Olympic athletes (Academic Press, New York 1974).

Jeurissen, A.: L'âge au moment des premières règles et son évolution en Belgique au cours des quarante dernières années. Acta paediat. belg. *23:* 319–330 (1969).

Jungman, H. (ed.): Sportwissenschaftliche Untersuchung während der XX. Olympischen Spiele, München 1972 (Demeter, Gräfeling 1976).

Kohlrausch, W.: Zusammenhang von Körperform und Leistung. Arbeitsphysiol. *2:* 187–204 (1929).

Lopez, A.; Rojas, J.; Garcia, E.: Somatotype et composition du corps chez les gymnastes de haut niveau. Cinésiol. *18:* 5–18 (1979).

Maas, G.D.: The physique of athletes. An anthropometric study of 285 top sportsmen from 14 sports in a total of 774 athletes (Leiden University Press, Leiden 1974).

Malina, R.M.: A multidisciplinary, biocultural approach to physical performance; in Ostyn, Beunen, Simons, Kinanthropometry II, Int. Ser. Sport Scienc., vol. IX, pp. 33–68 (University Park Press, Baltimore 1980).

Märker, K.: Zur Menarche von Sportlerinnen nach mehrjährigem Training im Kindesalter. Med. Sport *19:* 329–332 (1979).

Novotny, V.V.; Taftlova, R.: Biological age and sport fitness of young gymnast women; in Novotny, Anthropological Congr., pp. 123–130 (Czechoslovak Academy of Sciences, Prague 1971).

Parizkova, J.: Body fat and physical fitness (Nijhoff, The Hague 1977).

Roche, A.F.: Secular trends in stature, weight and maturation; in Roche, Secular trends in human growth, maturation, and development. Monogr. Soc. Res. Child Dev. *179:* 3–27 (1979).

Simons, J.; Beunen, G.; Ostyn, M.; Renson, R.; Swalus, P.; Gerven, D. van; Willems, E.:
Construction d'une batterie de tests d'aptitude motrice pour garçons de 12 à 19 ans
par la méthode d'analyse factorielle. Kinanthrop. *1:* 323–362 (1969).

Sinning, W.E.; Lindberg, G.D.: Physical characteristics of college age women gymnasts
Res. Quart. *43:* 226–234 (1972).

Stepnicka, J.: Typological and motor characteristics of athletes and university students
(in Czech) (Charles University, Prague 1972).

Tanner, J.M.: The physique of the Olympic athlete (Allen & Unwin, London 1964).

Tanner, J.M.; Whitehouse, R.H.; Marshall, W.A.; Healy, M.J.R.; Goldstein, H.: Assessment of skeletal maturity and prediction of adult height (TW2 method) (Academic
Press, London 1975).

Tittel, K.: Zur Biotypologie und funktionellen Anatomie des Leistungssportlers. Nova
Acta Leopoldina, vol. 30 (Barth, Leipzig 1968).

Tittel, K.; Wutscherk, H.: Sportanthropometrie (Barth, Leipzig 1972).

Wilmore, J.: The application of science to sport: physiological profiles of male and female
athletes. Can. J. appl. Sport Sci. *4:* 103–118 (1979).

Zaharieva, E.; Georgiev, N.; Tchechmedgiev, R.: Recherches anthropométriques sur
les gymnastes masculins et féminins des XVIIIe championnats du monde de Varna
(Bulgarie) de 1974. Cinésiol. *18:* 19–24 (1979).

Dr. G. Beunen, K.U. Leuven, Institute of Physical Education,
Tervuurse Vest 101, B-3030 Heverlee (Belgium)

Medicine Sport, vol. 15, pp. 186–191 (Karger, Basel 1981)

Physique of College Women Athletes in Five Sports

M.H. Slaughter, T.G. Lohman, R.A. Boileau, W.F. Riner

Physical Fitness Research Laboratory, Department of Physical Education,
University of Illinois, Urbana-Champaign, Ill., USA

Introduction

It is well known that athletes participating in different sports and in different events or positions within the same sport vary in physique. *Tanner et al.* [1980] indicated that physique and body composition to a large extent predispose individuals to certain types of athletic ability. *Carter* [1970] has raised several key questions regarding physique of athletes including the one which asks: 'If physique and physical performance are related, at what level of competition does this selective factor become recognizable?' Although several studies on the physique of athletes have been conducted on both sexes at high levels of competition, research on the relation of physique to sport in female college athletes is lacking.

The purpose of this study was to determine differences in body size, composition and structure among 5 women athletic teams and to compare the differences in relative musculo-skeletal development using an objective method for characterizing body physique using fat-free body weight (estimated from underwater weighing) in relation to height.

Procedure

The subjects in this study included 63 members of the University of Illinois women's athletic teams, including 16 swimmers, 13 gymnasts, 12 tennis players, 11 cross-country runners, and 11 track and field participants. The track and field group were made up of long jumpers, sprinters, high jumpers, hurdlers, 440-yard runners, a shot putter and a discus thrower. The average age for the athletes was 19.8 years, ranging from 17.8 to 22.5.

They ranged in height from 152.7 to 182.0 cm, with a mean of 164.8 cm and ranged in weight from 45.6 to 82.3 kg, with a mean of 52.9 kg.

Body density (Db) was measured by underwater weighing [*Buskirk*, 1961] with procedures and instrumentation modified according to *Akers and Buskirk* [1969]. Further details of this procedure are given in *Lohman* et al. [1978]. Relative body fatness (percentage fat) was computed from body density accordingly [*Brozek* et al., 1963]: percentage fat = $(4.570/D - 4 \cdot 142) \times 100$.

The anthropometric dimensions included six skinfold sites, seven girth, and six skeletal widths. Three consecutive measurements were taken at each site on each of 2 days and the mean of the three measurements for each day was used at the measurement for a given site. All skinfold thickness measurements were made with a Harpenden caliper on the right side of the body. The skinfolds measured were triceps, subscapular suprailiac, abdominal, midaxillary, and medial calf. The girths measured were biceps (flexed), forearm girth, minimum wrist girth of the forearm, thigh girth, calf girth, ankle girth, chest girth inflated and deflated. Skeletal widths included biepicondylar breadth of the humerus, wrist width (taken between styloid process of radius and ulnar), biepicondylar breadth of the femur, ankle breadth (taken between malleoli), biacromial breadth, and biilocristal breadth. All anthropometric dimensions are described by *Lohman* et al. [1978].

Results and Discussion

Means of selected physical characteristics for college women athletes in five sports are presented in table I along with 'F' ratios and results of Duncan's post hoc tests. On height the group means for the swimming (170.1 cm) and track teams (167.1 cm) were significantly higher than the other three groups, but did not differ significantly from each other. In terms of weight the mean for the swimmers (64.0 kg) was significantly heavier than the other four groups, with track (57.7 kg) and tennis (57.7 kg) the next heaviest, though not significantly different from each other. In terms of fat-free weight, the swimmers (47.9 kg), track (46.3 kg), and gymnasts (44.6 kg) had the greatest amount of fat-free weight and were significantly higher than the tennis (44.0 kg) and cross-country team (42.5 kg).

In terms of body composition, the swimming team (25.3%) had a significantly greater percent fat than the cross-country team (16.7%), track team (19.5%), and the gymnastic team (19.8%), but was not significantly different from the tennis team (24.7%).

For skinfolds, the swimming team had the highest measures in both back and side sites and the second largest in triceps, with the cross-country team having the lowest measures at all three sites. The swimming team differed significantly from the cross-country team (10.9 mm), gymnastic team (12.9 mm), and track team (13.5 mm), but did not differ from the

Table I. Means for selected physical characteristics of college women athletes in five sports, 'F' ratios and results of Duncan's post hoc tests[1,2]

	Track team	Gym-nastics team	Tennis team	Cross-country team	Swim team	F	Total group
Height, cm	167.1b	159.8a	162.8a	162.8a	170.1b	10.82^2	164.8
Weight, kg	57.7b	55.6a,b	58.6b	51.0a	64.0b,c	7.52^2	57.9
% fat	19.5a	19.8a	24.7b	16.7a	25.3b	9.75^2	21.6
Fat-free weight	46.3a,b	44.6a,b	44.0a	42.5a	46.3a,b	2.9	45.3
Biceps flexed girth, cm	25.1a,b	26.5b,c	26.0a,b,c	24.4a	27.7c	3.9^2	26.1
Calf girth, cm	33.3a	33.9a	34.3a,b	32.9a	35.7b	3.6^2	34.1
Biepicondylar breadth of humerus, cm	5.8a	5.8a	6.7b	5.7a	6.0a	13.36^2	6.0
Biepicondylar breadth of femur, cm	8.6c	7.4a	8.5b,c	8.3b,c	8.1b	7.21^2	8.1
Triceps skf, mm	13.5a	12.9a	17.4b	10.9a	16.4b	7.07^2	14.4
Subscapular skf, mm	10.0b	10.1b	10.2b	7.4a	11.3b	3.82^2	9.9
Suprailiac skf, mm	8.4a,b	10.5b	10.3b	6.7a	10.7b	4.07^2	9.5
Deviations from non-athletic line, kg	2.4a	4.3a	2.1a	0.59a	2.3a	1.19	2.3

[1] Group means with the same superscripts do not differ significantly from one another.
[2] $p < 0.05$.
[3] *Slaughter and Lohman* [1980].

tennis team (17.4 mm) on the triceps skinfold. The cross-country team was significantly lower than the other four teams (track, 10.0 mm; gymnastic, 10.1 mm; tennis 10.2 mm, and swimming 11.3 mm, respectively) on the sub-scapular skinfold. The suprailiac skinfold measure followed a similar though not identical pattern.

In terms of girths, the cross-country team had the smallest measure for both biceps flexed girths (24.4 cm) and calf girth (32.9 cm), while the swimming team had the largest girth measures with a 27.7 cm biceps flexed girth and a 35.7 cm calf girth. The cross-country team differed significantly from the track team (25.1 and 33.3 cm) and swimming team (27.4 and 35.7 cm) on both girths. The swimming team also differed (p 0.05) from the cross-country and track teams on the biceps flexed circumference and the gym-nastic (33.7 cm), cross-country (32.9 cm) and track teams (33.3 cm) on the calf girth.

In terms of skeletal width, in general, the tennis players and swimmers had the largest skeletal widths with the cross-country and gymnasts being the smallest. The tennis team had a significantly larger biepicondylar breadth of humerus (6.7 cm) than all other teams and both track (8.5 cm) and tennis team (6.7 cm) had a significantly greater biepicondylar breadth of the femur than gymnastic team (7.4 cm). The gymnastic (7.4 cm) team, moreover, had a significantly smaller biepicondylar breadth of the femur width than all other teams.

Thus, in general, it can be concluded that the tennis and swimming teams are the largest in terms of body size, and percent fat with the gymnastic and cross-country teams being the smallest.

It was of interest not only to compare the University of Illinois women athletic teams to each other on physique measurements, but also to see how these college athletes compared to top-level athletes. Illinois swimmers were taller than the Olympic swimmers of *Novak* et al. [1977] (170.1 cm as compared to 167.0 cm), weighed much more (64.0 kg as compared to 60.1 kg) and were fatter, 25.3% as compared to 18.9%.

The Illinois gymnasts were shorter than the Olympic gymnasts of *Novak* et al. [1977] (159.8 cm compared to 163.5 cm), weighed less, 51.0 kg compared to 52.5 cm, and were fatter (19.8% compared to 12.9%).

The Illinois cross-country team were shorter (162.8 cm as compared to 169.4 cm), weighed less (51.0 kg as compared to 57.2 kg), much fatter (167.7% as compared to 9.1%) and had less fat-free weight (42.5 kg as compared to 48.1 kg) than a group of national-class cross-country women [*Wilmore and Brown*, 1974].

Recently an objective method for studying the relation of fat-free body to height was proposed by *Slaughter and Lohman* [1980] and the application of this method for the 5 women athletic teams is shown in figure 1. The authors propose that the regression of FFB on height be used as a method for evaluating the relative musculo-skeletal size in athletes. The regression of FFB on height is proposed as a method of evaluating relative musculo-skeletal size rather than FFB/ht since implicit in the use of this ratio is the assumption that the underlying relation between FFB and height is a straight line with a slope equal to the mean FFB over the mean height and an intercept of zero. Previous work indicated that the intercept was not zero and the slope was better estimated by a regression equation [*Slaughter and Lohman*, unpublished]. The extent to which one falls above or below the regression line is proposed as an index of musculo-skeletal size. For the athletic groups the mean deviation (kg) from the non-athletic line ranged from 0.59 kg (0.2 SEE above the regression line) for the cross-country team to a high of 4.3 kg for the gymnastic team (1.2 SEE above the regression

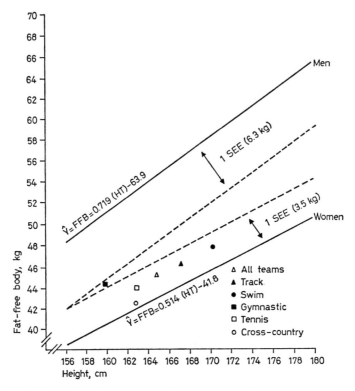

Fig. 1. Deviations from the non-athletic regression line of FFB on height in college women athletes.

line). Thus, in terms of musculo-skeletal size, the gymnastic team had the greatest amount of fat-free weight in relation to size, while the cross-country team had the least. Many more athletic teams need to be measured before a true assessment of the importance of this index is understood.

Summary

The purpose of this study was to determine differences in body size, composition, and structure, among 5 women athletic teams, and to compare the differences in relative musculo-skeletal development using an objective method for characterizing body physique using fat-free body in relation to height.

Significant differences in body size, composition and structure were found as well as differences between deviation scores among the five athletic teams.

References

Akers, R.; Buskirk, E.R.: An underwater weighing system utilizing force cube transducers. J. appl. Physiol. *26:* 649–652 (1969).

Brozek, J.; Grande, J.T.; Anderson, T.; Keys, A.: Densitometric analysis of body composition: a revision of some quantitative assumptions. Ann. N.Y. Acad. Sci. *110:* 113–140 (1963).

Buskirk, E.R.: Underwater weighing and body density: a review of procedures; in Brozek, Techniques for measuring body composition of procedures (Natn. Academy of Science, Washington 1961).

Carter, J.E.L.: The somatotype of athletes – a review. Hum. Biol. *42:* 535–569 (1970).

Lohman, T.G.; Slaughter, M.H.; Selinger, A.; Boileau, R.A.: Relationship of body composition to somatotype in college men. Annals Human Biol. *5:* 147–157 (1978).

Novak, L.P.; Woodmar, W.A.; Bestil, C.; Mellorowicz, H.: Working capacity body composition and anthropometry of Olympic female athletes. J. Sports Med. phys. Fit. *17:* 275–283 (1977).

Slaughter, M.H.; Lohman, T.G.: An objective method for measurement of musculoskeletal size to characterize body physique with application to the athletic population. Med. Sci. Sports *12:* 174–178 (1980).

Tanner, J.M.; Israelsohn, W.J.; Whitehouse, R.H.: Physique and body composition as factors affecting success in different athletic events. Med. Sportiva *14:* 397–411 (1980).

Wilmore, J.H.; Brown, C.H.: Physiological profiles of women distance runners. Medicine Sci. Sport *6:* 178–181 (1974).

Dr. M.H. Slaughter, Physical Fitness Research Laboratory, Department of Physical Education, University of Illinois, Urbana-Champaign, IL 61820 (USA)

Medicine Sport, vol. 15, pp. 192–200 (Karger, Basel 1981)

Measures of Body Size and Form of Elite Female Basketball Players

J.H. Spurgeon, N.L. Spurgeon, W.K. Giese

Department of Physical Education, University of South Carolina, Columbia, S.C., USA

Introduction

Certainly in the United States, and to a varying extent elsewhere, the development and expansion of opportunity in girls' and women's sports in the decade of the seventies was unprecedented. Facilities, funds, and opportunities to compete make possible investigations previously confined to male competitors.

Purpose

This is a descriptive and comparative report on the physique of world-class Bulgarian, Canadian, Czechoslovakian, Polish, Russian, and United States female basketball players. Data were gathered partly in December 1978 at Columbia, S.C., and partly in August 1979 at Squaw Valley, Calif. In both instances the anthropometrist was the same.

Results and Discussion

The subjects were 84 females, each of whom was a current or former member of a national team, national championship team, Olympic team, All-American team, or participant on one or more international teams in competition such as the Pan-American Games, Spartaciade, Summer Sports Festival, World University Games, or European championship. In respect to basketball-playing positions, there were 21 centers, 31 forwards, and 32 guards: some subjects, of course, played in more than one position, but these were the primary positions listed by the head coach of each team. 78 subjects were Caucasian, and 6 were of Negroid ancestry. Average age was 22.1 years.

Data were obtained for 11 measures of body size (standing height, sitting height, upper limb length, lower limb length, arm girth, shoulder width, hip width, chest girth, abdomen girth, leg girth, and body weight); 7 indices of body form (lower limb length/sitting height (skelic index), hip width/shoulder width (trunk width index I), $3 \times$ shoulder width minus hip width (trunk width index II), chest girth/abdomen girth, chest girth/standing height, calf girth/lower limb length, and arm girth/arm length); and a measure of body composition. The procedure for measures of body size is described by *Spurgeon and Meredith* [1978], and that for body composition by *Sloan* et al. [1962].

Tables I and II display the means for measures of body size, body form, and body composition for each of the national groups of world-class female basketball players. The following are examples of the many descriptions that can be extracted from these tables: (1) The Czechoslovakian team is tallest and the Bulgarian team shortest, with a difference of almost 5.0 cm. Incidentally, the girls who measured above 183 cm had been told they were taller than our records showed by 3.0 cm or more. It is not known whether they had been incorrectly measured, measured wearing shoes, or misinformed. (2) Means for sitting height vary from near 92 cm for the USA team to near 94 cm for the Czechoslovakian team. Means for arm girth are near 27 cm for the Bulgarian, Canadian, Polish, and USA teams. (3) The skelic index is near 89 for the Bulgarian team, near 92 for the Polish and USSR teams, and near 93 for the Canadian, Czechoslovakian, and USA teams. Comparatively, the Czechoslovakian and USA teams have narrow hips relative to shoulder width (trunk width index I), while the Bulgarian and USSR teams have wide hips relative to shoulder width. (4) Teams were remarkably alike in estimated percentage of body fat. Low body fat is associated with high fitness [*Spurgeon* et al., 1978]. Consequently, 17–18% body fat can be taken to characterize female basketball players of world-class ability and fitness.

Tables III and IV present the means for measures of body size, body form, and body composition, by team position, for the 6 national groups of world-class female basketball players studied. It is found: (1) For each national group, in standing height and body weight the centers surpass the forwards, and the forwards surpass the guards. (2) Except for the Czecho-

Table I. Means for measures of the body size of 84 world-class female basketball players

Measurement[1]	Bulgaria	Canada	Czecho-slovakia	Poland	USSR	US	Total
Standing height	176.8	180.7	181.7	178.1	180.4	178.4	179.2
Sitting height	93.5	93.5	94.2	93.0	93.7	92.3	93.2
Upper limb length	76.4	78.5	–	76.7	77.7	74.8	76.5
Lower limb length	83.3	87.2	87.5	85.1	86.6	86.0	86.0
Shoulder width	39.7	38.9	38.1	38.6	39.3	38.0	38.6
Hip width	31.7	30.6	29.1	29.7	31.9	28.7	30.1
Chest girth	80.1	80.2	–	79.5	81.7	78.7	79.8
Abdomen girth	83.6	79.3	–	81.8	84.5	79.9	81.5
Arm girth	27.3	27.2	–	27.3	28.1	27.2	27.4
Calf girth	36.2	37.8	–	37.8	37.5	36.9	37.2
Body weight	69.0	70.7	70.2	69.9	74.0	68.7	70.1
Number of women	12	12	12	12	12	24	84

[1] Body weight in kilograms and all other values in centimeters.

Table II. Means for measures of the body form and body composition of 84 world-class female basketball players

Index	Bulgaria	Canada	Czecho-slovakia	Poland	USSR	US	Total
Skelic index	89.1	93.3	92.8	91.6	92.4	93.3	92.2
Trunk width index I	79.9	78.6	76.3	77.0	81.2	76.4	78.0
Trunk width index II	87.3	86.1	85.3	86.2	85.9	85.1	85.7
Trunk girth index	96.0	101.3	–	97.2	96.9	98.1	97.9
Chest-height index	45.4	44.4	–	44.7	45.4	44.2	44.7
Lower limb index	43.6	43.3	–	44.6	43.4	42.9	43.5
Upper limb index	35.8	34.7	–	35.6	36.2	35.1	35.4
Fat, %	17.7	17.7	–	17.9	17.9	17.2	17.6
Number of women	12	12	12	12	12	24	84

slovakian and USA teams, the skelic index means decrease from centers to forwards and from forwards to guards. Among the USA team, 4 of the 12 forwards were of Negroid ancestry. Negroid and Caucasoid groups differ markedly in mean skelic index [*Meredith and Spurgeon*, 1976]. (3) For each national group, centers exceed guards in trunk width index II. In each of the 5 groups on which upper and lower limb indices were derived, guards

Table III. Means for eleven measures of body size for world-class female basketball players for six nations

National group and positions	n	Standing height	Sitting height	Upper limb length	Lower limb length	Shoulder width	Hip width	Chest girth	Abdomen girth	Arm girth	Calf girth	Body weight
Bulgaria	12											
Centers	3	185.0	97.0	81.0	88.0	40.5	32.6	85.3	87.0	27.7	38.3	77.5
Forwards	4	179.6	94.3	76.9	85.3	39.8	32.9	78.6	82.8	26.7	36.3	68.5
Guards	5	169.6	90.7	73.2	78.9	39.0	30.2	79.4	82.2	27.5	35.0	64.2
Canada	12											
Centers	4	187.9	95.2	82.5	92.7	39.7	31.0	81.3	81.4	27.9	38.9	77.5
Forwards	3	181.5	94.8	78.9	86.7	39.9	32.6	84.9	82.3	27.8	38.7	75.6
Guards	5	174.4	91.3	75.1	83.1	37.6	29.1	76.5	75.8	26.4	36.2	62.2
Czechoslovakia	12											
Centers	5	189.8	97.9	–	92.0	39.2	30.3	–	–	–	–	78.4
Forwards	3	184.1	93.7	–	90.4	38.4	29.8	–	–	–	–	71.3
Guards	4	169.8	90.1	–	79.7	36.6	27.2	–	–	–	–	59.1
Poland	12											
Centers	3	183.4	94.3	79.2	89.1	40.8	31.3	79.5	85.6	27.8	39.2	74.9
Forwards	4	182.7	96.2	79.3	86.5	38.7	30.2	82.3	84.5	27.9	38.5	74.2
Guards	5	171.0	89.7	73.6	81.5	37.3	28.3	77.2	77.4	26.4	36.4	63.5
Soviet Union	12											
Centers	2	190.9	98.0	81.1	93.0	40.7	32.8	86.6	89.3	29.6	39.7	87.0
Forwards	5	185.7	96.0	80.8	89.8	40.7	34.4	81.8	85.7	27.7	38.2	77.0
Guards	5	170.7	89.8	73.3	80.9	37.2	29.1	79.6	81.3	27.9	35.9	65.8
United States	24											
Centers	4	187.0	96.2	81.6	90.8	38.8	29.6	80.5	83.1	27.8	37.4	73.7
Forwards	12	180.8	93.8	79.3	88.1	38.4	29.0	79.1	81.4	27.4	37.5	71.6
Guards	8	170.4	89.9	73.5	80.5	36.8	27.9	77.3	76.2	26.6	35.6	61.7

Table IV. Means for seven measures of body form and one measure of body composition for world-class female basketball players of six nations

National group and positions	n	Skelic index	Trunk width index I	Trunk width index II	Trunk girth index	Chest height index	Lower limb index	Upper limb index	Fat % body weight
Bulgaria	12								
Centers	3	90.7	80.6	89.0	96.0	45.1	43.5	34.3	17.1
Forwards	4	90.5	82.8	86.5	95.1	43.8	42.7	34.7	15.4
Guards	5	87.0	77.3	87.0	96.6	46.8	44.4	37.6	19.8
Canada	12								
Centers	4	97.6	77.9	88.2	99.8	43.2	42.0	34.1	19.1
Forwards	3	91.5	81.6	87.2	103.6	46.8	44.6	35.2	19.9
Guards	5	91.0	77.5	83.7	101.1	43.9	43.6	35.1	15.4
Czechoslovakia	12								
Centers	5	94.0	77.2	87.4	–	–	–	–	–
Forwards	3	96.5	77.6	85.3	–	–	–	–	–
Guards	4	88.4	74.3	82.7	–	–	–	–	–
Poland	12								
Centers	3	94.5	76.9	91.0	92.8	43.4	44.0	35.2	18.9
Forwards	4	90.1	78.1	85.9	97.4	45.0	44.6	35.2	20.1
Guards	5	87.0	77.3	87.0	96.6	45.2	44.9	36.2	15.5
Soviet Union	12								
Centers	2	95.0	80.7	89.2	97.0	45.4	42.7	36.5	17.0
Forwards	5	93.6	84.6	87.9	95.6	44.0	42.7	34.3	17.7
Guards	5	90.2	78.1	82.6	98.1	46.7	44.5	38.1	18.5
United States	24								
Centers	4	94.6	76.4	86.8	96.9	43.0	41.3	34.0	18.1
Forwards	12	95.2	76.8	86.4	96.4	43.7	42.6	34.7	17.1
Guards	8	89.7	75.8	82.5	101.6	45.4	44.2	36.3	16.9

surpass centers in limb stockiness. Trunk girth relative to abdominal girth is higher for guards than centers of the Canadian, Polish, USSR and USA teams.

In tables V and VI the national groups are combined and, at each playing position, means and variability values are given for measures of body size, body form, and body composition, are as follows: (1) In all measures of body size, centers are largest, followed by forwards, then guards. On the whole, there is greater difference between centers and forwards than between forwards and guards. This is as expected since centers and forwards play near the basket where size, strength, and jumping ability are advantageous. (2) The greatest variability found among measures of body size is

Table V. Means and variability statistics for eleven measures of body size on world-class female basketball centers, forwards, and guards

Position	n	Mean	SD	Minimum	Maximum
Standing height					
Centers	21	187.0	4.1	180.5	196.7
Forwards	31	182.1	3.4	174.0	188.8
Guards	32	171.0	3.2	163.5	176.5
Sitting height					
Centers	21	96.4	2.7	89.7	101.3
Forwards	31	94.2	2.8	86.3	101.0
Guards	32	90.2	1.8	86.0	93.1
Upper limb length					
Centers	16	81.2	2.8	76.4	87.7
Forwards	28	79.2	2.0	74.7	83.3
Guards	28	73.7	2.4	69.2	77.3
Lower limb length					
Centers	21	91.0	3.4	84.4	97.5
Forwards	31	87.9	3.5	80.9	97.1
Guards	32	80.8	3.0	73.2	84.7
Shoulder width					
Centers	21	39.8	1.5	36.9	43.0
Forwards	31	39.2	1.6	36.1	42.9
Guards	32	37.4	1.5	34.6	40.7
Hip width					
Centers	21	31.0	1.7	28.8	35.2
Forwards	31	30.9	3.0	26.8	37.7
Guards	32	28.6	1.5	25.6	31.6
Chest girth					
Centers	16	81.8	4.1	73.9	86.9
Forwards	28	80.6	2.9	75.1	85.8
Guards	28	77.9	2.6	73.1	82.6
Abdomen girth					
Centers	16	84.6	4.4	77.3	91.9
Forwards	28	82.9	4.8	72.1	93.8
Guards	28	78.3	4.2	69.8	86.9
Arm girth					
Centers	16	28.0	2.0	23.9	32.0
Forwards	28	27.5	1.2	25.3	29.7
Guards	28	26.9	1.4	24.3	30.3
Calf girth					
Centers	16	38.6	2.5	35.8	44.4
Forwards	28	37.7	1.5	35.0	41.0
Guards	28	35.8	1.7	33.0	41.1

Table V. Continued

Position	n	Mean	SD	Minimum	Maximum
Body weight					
Centers	21	77.5	6.9	62.9	89.5
Forwards	31	72.8	4.8	63.7	81.9
Guards	32	62.8	4.2	56.4	75.0

in body weight. The range among centers extends from the tall and moderately linear performer to the tall and moderately stocky performer. This is reflected in body composition. (3) The means for the skelic index are from 6 to 8% higher than would be expected in the female population in general [*Spurgeon and Meredith*, 1979]. The index is especially high among centers and forwards where jumping ability for rebounding is vital. For two women of the same height, the women with the greater skelic index (greater lower limb length relative to sitting height) would be expected to jump higher because her crotch is farther above the ground. (4) As has been documented by many [*Carter*, 1970; *de Garay* et al., 1974; *Eiben*, 1969, 1972; *Malina* et al., 1971; *Malina and Zavaleta*, 1976; *Tanner*, 1964] and inferred in this study, athletes participating in different sports, and those participating in different events or positions within the same sport, differ in size and physique. Just as track and field jumpers and hurdlers differ from throwers, so do participants at different positions in basketball. In all probability most female athletes have a somewhat more masculine appearing physique than is typical of the female population in general. The two indexes reflecting physique masculinity are trunk width indexes I and II. While the indexes serve different functions and are not directly comparable there is a moderate inverse relation between them. A low trunk width index I score or a high trunk width index II score would provide the visual 'V' impression that is characteristic of some mesomorphs. It is apparent that some very powerful and physically masculine women are included among these female basketball players, especially the centers and forwards. In comparison with the 1968 Mexican Olympic findings [*de Garay* et al., 1974], the guards are similar to sprinters (84.3) and the forwards and centers compare closely to jumpers (85.2) and javelin throwers (87.8). There appears to be considerable overlap in trunk width index II scores among participants from sport to sport, and from position to position within sports. If the trunk width index II scores had

Table VI. Means and variability statistics for seven measures of body form and one measure of body composition for world-class female basketball centers, forwards, and guards

Position	n	Means	SD	Minimum	Maximum
Skelic index					
Centers	21	94.5	4.5	85.3	102.1
Forwards	31	93.4	5.6	81.7	112.5
Guards	32	89.6	4.1	81.1	97.6
Trunk width index I					
Centers	21	77.9	5.2	71.6	86.9
Forwards	31	79.5	7.4	69.3	96.9
Guards	32	76.5	3.5	69.0	84.2
Trunk width index II					
Centers	16	88.3	3.9	80.9	98.2
Forwards	28	86.5	4.5	77.8	98.2
Guards	28	83.6	3.8	77.6	91.6
Trunk girth index					
Centers	16	96.7	3.5	88.9	100.9
Forwards	28	97.0	6.7	77.7	108.9
Guards	28	99.7	3.9	94.1	111.5
Chest height index					
Centers	16	43.8	2.0	40.6	47.9
Forwards	28	44.3	1.7	40.4	48.0
Guards	28	45.6	2.0	41.6	49.5
Lower limb index					
Centers	16	42.6	3.2	38.8	51.1
Forwards	28	43.1	2.5	37.6	49.7
Guards	28	44.3	2.6	40.1	50.0
Upper limb index					
Centers	16	34.6	3.0	29.1	41.2
Forwards	28	34.7	1.6	32.1	38.0
Guards	28	36.6	2.5	32.9	41.9
Fat, % body weight					
Centers	16	18.2	2.9	14.1	23.8
Forwards	28	17.7	3.4	13.3	27.5
Guards	28	17.2	2.5	13.0	24.0

been ample to determine their predictive value in sports participation, this would have been helpful to coaches. At this junctive, however, further research on the matter is needed. As women's sports, and the number of women participating, continue to grow, and larger data pools become available, it likely will become possible to develop useful predictive procedures.

Summary

The subjects were 84 world-class female basketball players on national teams of Bulgaria, Canada, Czechoslovakia, Poland, Soviet Union, and United States. Measures were taken of standing and sitting height, upper and lower limb length, shoulder and hip width, chest and abdomen girth, arm and calf girth, and body weight. Body form was studied using indices of lower limb to sitting height, shoulder to hip width, chest to abdomen girth, and limb girth to limb length. Averages and variability statistics are presented. Relative comparisons are made between national groups and playing positions. The USSR team is heaviest, the Czechoslovak team tallest. Skelic index is highest for centers, lowest for guards. The percent body fat was similar for all teams and, within teams, the lowest for the guards.

References

Carter, J.E.L.: The somatotype of athletes – a review. Hum. Biol. 42: 535–569 (1970).
Eiben, O.: Konstitutionsbiologische Untersuchungen an europäischen Hochleistungs-sportlerinnen. Wiss. Z. Humboldt Univ. Berlin, Math.-Nat. R 18: 941–946 (1969)
Eiben, O.: The physique of women athletes, pp. 1–190 (Hungarian Scientific Council for Physical Education, Budapest 1972).
Garay, A.L. de; Levine, L.; Carter, J.E.L.: Genetic and anthropological studies of Olympic athletes, pp. 1–236 (Academic Press, New York 1974).
Malina, R.M.; Harper, A.B.; Avent, H.H.; Campbell, D.E.: Physique of female track and field athletes. Med. Sci. Sports 3: 32–38 (1971).
Malina, R.M.; Zavaleta, A.N.: Androgyny of physique in female track and field athletes. Ann. hum. Biol. 3: 441–446 (1976).
Meredith, H.V.; Spurgeon, J.H.: Comparative findings on the skelic index of black and white children and youths residing in South Carolina. Growth 40: 75–81 (1976).
Sloan, A.W.; Burt, J.J.; Blyth, C.S.: Estimation of body fat in young women. J. appl. Physiol. 17: 967–970 (1962).
Spurgeon, J.H.; Blair, S.N.; Keith, J.A.; McGinn, C.J.: Characteristics of successful and probationary high school football officials. Phys. Sports Med. 6: 106–112 (1978).
Spurgeon, J.H.; Meredith, H.V.: Body size and form of children of predominantly black ancestry living in West and Central Africa, North and South America, and the West Indies. Ann. hum. Biol. 5: 229–246 (1978).
Spurgeon, J.H.; Meredith, H.V.: Secular change of body size and form of black American children and youths living in the United States. Paper presented 2nd Int. Symp. of Human Biology, Visegrad 1979.
Tanner, J.M.: The physique of the Olympic athlete, pp. 1–126 (Allen & Unwin, London 1964).

Prof. Dr. John H. Spurgeon, Blatt Physical Education Center, University of South Carolina, Columbia, SC 29208 (USA)

Medicine Sport, vol. 15, pp. 201–205 (Karger, Basel 1981)

Body Build of Female Olympic Rowers

M. Hebbelinck, W.D. Ross, J.E.L. Carter, J. Borms

Vrije Universiteit Brussel, Laboratory of Human Biometry and Biomechanics, HILOK, Brussels, Belgium; Simon Fraser University, Department of Kinesiology, Burnaby, B.C., Canada; San Diego State University, Department of Physical Education, San Diego, Calif., USA

Rowing for women is a new sport at the Olympics, being first admitted at the 1976 Montreal Olympic Games. While structural and functional studies have been made on male Olympic and other groups of elite rowers, there have been few studies on female elite rowers [*Parnell*, 1951; *Titlbachova*, 1972]. The occasion of the Montreal Olympic Games, therefore, provided an opportunity to assemble data on some of the best female rowers in the world.

The purpose of this paper was to provide a description of certain anthropometric characteristics of female Olympic rowers.

Subjects

The Olympic rowers in this study were volunteers who responded to an invitation to participate as subjects in the Montreal Olympic Games Anthropological Project (MOGAP). This procedure was perhaps biased, in that the act of coming to the laboratories of the Olympic Village was a result of various influences and motives.

The MOGAP sample (table I) consisted of 51 rowers out of a total of 223 female rowers, i.e. 23%, excluding coxwains. 38 (75%) of the subjects were from Canada or the United States of America. The remainder were from Europe (Netherlands, Great Britain, Norway and Czechoslovakia). The sample included one silver medalist, 8 bronze medalists and 15 other finalists. Thus, roughly half the sample were finalists.

Anthropometric Measurements

The anthropometric measurements have been reported by *Borms* et al. [1979]. The variables measured included heights and lengths, breadths, girths, skinfolds, age and weight.

Table I. Number of female rowers by event and geographic region (Montreal Olympic Games, 1976)

Event	North America	Europe	Totals
Single sculls	2	–	2
Double sculls	2	2	4
Pairs without cox	2	4	6
Fours with cox	6	1	7
Quad sculls with cox	8	1	9
Eights with cox	18	5	23
Totals	38	13	51
Scullers[1]	12	3	15
Sweepers[2]	26	10	36

[1] Scullers = single, double and quad sculls. [2] Sweepers = pairs, fours and eights.

Results and Discussion

The representativeness of the rower sample of 51 compared to the overall group of 223 female rowers participating in the Montreal Games was inferred by a t-test for height and weight data reported at registration. As shown in table II, the sample of 51 were not significantly different in height from the remaining 172 female rowers. However, they were significantly lighter (–3.1 kg).

Reported measures of height and weight at registration are somewhat suspect. Moreover, there may have been a change in weight between the time of registration and the time of measurement. As shown in table III, a comparison of reported and obtained height and weight showed no significant difference in height; however, there was a small but significant difference in weight (+1.6 kg) for the 51 female rowers of the MOGAP sample.

Descriptive statistics of age and 30 anthropometric measures are summarized in table IV; comparisons were made in percentiles with other female athletes of the Mexico Olympic Games [*Carter* et al., 1978] and in T-scores with a reference group of female Canadian university students.

The mean T-scores was 61.6 for the heights, lengths, breadths and girths. In normally distributed data this would be at the 94th percentile level and would emphasize the rowers' comparatively greater size than nonrowers. The mean T-score was 44.0 for the skinfold thicknesses which in

Table II. Comparison of reported height and weight (mean and standard deviation) at registration by MOGAP sample and that reported by the remainder of the female rowers (Montreal Olympic Games, 1976)

	MOGAP (n = 51)	Remainder (N-n = 172)	Difference	t-ratio
Height, cm	174.3	175.1	-0.8	-1.06
	(4.71)	(4.88)		
Weight, kg	67.4	70.5	-3.1	-2.30*
	(5.28)	(7.42)		

* Significant at the 0.05 level.

Table III. Comparison of reported and obtained height and weight values (mean and standard deviation) for MOGAP female Olympic rowers (n = 51)

	Obtained at MOGAP	Reported at registration	Difference	Wilcoxon's z-value
Height, cm	174.3	174.0	0.3	-0.937
	(4.71)	(6.05)		
Weight, kg	67.4	65.8	1.6	-4.51*
	(5.28)	(6.06)		

* Significant at the 0.01 level.

normally distributed data would be at the 27th percentile level, and would emphasize the comparative leanness of the rowers.

When rowers were compared with other female Olympic athletes whose size values were displayed on a percentile table, it was evident that the percentile score of the female rowers were larger than the 50th percentile of the athletic group, except for the suprailiac skinfold, which was at the 46th percentile.

Compared to the scarce data on female rowers in the literature, the rowers in this study were taller and heavier. *Parnell* [1951] reported some anthropometric data on 18 members of the Oxford University Women's Rowing Club. The Oxford women's mean values were 8.2 cm shorter and 7.1 kg lighter than the MOGAP rowers.

Tittel and Wutscherk [1972] reported data assembled by *Titlbachova* prior to 1960, which showed Czechoslovakian women rowers to be 10.6 cm

Table IV. The means of anthropometric measures shown as T-scores of a non-rowers sample and as percentiles of the Mexico female Olympic athletes sample

Variables	Rowers (n=51)		T-Score ref. group	Percentile Olympic athletes
	x̄	SD		
Age, years	23.8	2.65	63	84
Weight, kg	67.4	5.33	66	87
Height and lengths, cm				
Height	174.3	4.78	64	87
Sitting	92.1	1.48	63	95
Upper arm	33.0	1.56	69	–
Forearm	23.9	1.15	58	–
Upper extremity	76.0	2.75	61	–
Upper extremity	56.9	2.29	61	70
Ilio-spinal	96.5	4.11	63	–
Foot	25.4	1.09	65	–
Breadths, cm				
Biacromial	37.4	1.46	62	60
Biiliocristal	28.2	1.79	54	75
Transverse chest	26.5	0.93	65	90
Anterior-posterior chest	18.1	1.32	58	65
Biepicondylar humerus	6.7	0.30	62	95
Biepicondylar femur	9.3	0.37	59	80
Girths, cm				
Arm girth flexed and contracted	29.3	1.56	64	76
Arm girth relaxed	27.6	1.48	59	86
Forearm girth (maximum relaxed)	25.5	0.99	63	–
Wrist girth (prox. styloid)	15.9	0.77	64	–
Chest girth (mesosternal)	89.6	3.45	61	–
Waist girth (minimum)	70.8	3.01	57	–
Thigh girth	57.5	2.94	56	85
Calf girth	37.0	1.62	61	85
Skinfolds, mm				
Triceps	14.6	4.07	45	85
Subscapular	9.1	2.69	44	57
Suprailiac	6.6	2.56	43	46
Umbilical	10.6	4.74	42	–
Front thigh	21.5	5.69	44	–
Medial calf	12.8	4.25	46	77
Triceps+subscapular+suprailiac	30.3	1.60	–	66

shorter and 4.3 kg lighter than the MOGAP sample. However, the data from both of these studies are dated and perhaps the subjects were not of the modern Olympic calibre of the MOGAP rowers.

Summary

Anthropometric data on 51 (23% of total group) of the female rowers in the 1976 Montreal Olympic Games are summarized and compared to a female non-rower athletic sample and to a female Canadian University student sample. The rowers, being taller and heavier (174.3 cm and 64 kg), tended to be larger in all 29 body measures than the reference samples with the exception of the university students, who had larger mean skinfold thicknesses.

References

Borms, J.; Hebbelinck, M.; Carter, J.E.L.; Ross, W.D.; Yuhasz, M.S.; Lariviere, G.: Standardization of basic anthropometry in Olympic athletes – the MOGAP procedure; in Novotny, Titlbachova, Methods of Functional Anthropology, Prague 1977, pp. 31–39 (Universitas Carolina, Prague 1979).

Carter, J.E.L.; Hebbelinck, M.; Garay, A.L. de: Anthropometric profiles of Olympic athletes at Mexico City; in Landry, Orban, Biomechanics of sports and kinanthropometry. Int. Congr. of Physical Activity Sciences, vol. 6, pp. 305–313 (Symposia Specialists, Miami 1978).

Parnell, R.W.: Some notes on physique and athletic training. Br. med. J. *1292:* 1–11 (1951).

Titlbachova, S.: cited in Tittel, Wutscherk, Sportanthropometrie, pp. 177–180 (Barth, Leipzig 1972).

Prof. Dr. M. Hebbelinck, Vrije Universiteit Brussel, Laboratory of Human Biometry and Biomechanics, HILOK, Pleinlaan 2, B-1050 Brussels (Belgium)

Biomechanics

Medicine Sport, vol. 15, pp. 206–215 (Karger, Basel 1981)

Body Segment Contributions of Female Athletes to Translational and Rotational Requirements of Non-Twisting Springboard Dive Takeoffs[1]

D.I. Miller

Department of Kinesiology, University of Washington, Seattle, Wash., USA

Introduction

In springboard diving, the athlete is projected into the air and must accomplish specific translational and rotational requirements. Since the influence of air resistance is minimal, the characteristics of the flight upon which the success or failure of the performance is usually judged, are predominantly predetermined by the diver's linear momentum and angular momentum when leaving the board. While adjustments can be made in the rate of spin or twist while in the air, the key to a successful performance lies in the takeoff preceding the flight. However, with the exception of some research providing limited information on body positions at touchdown, maximum board depression and final contact [*Miller*, 1974] and exemplary reaction force data from a Kistler platform mounted on a springboard [*Bergmaier*, 1970; *Bergmaier* et al., 1979], studies have not focused upon the mechanics of the springboard takeoff in a comprehensive and systematic manner. Further, most textbooks while acknowledging the importance of the takeoff, fail to provide much more than two or three illustrations of sequential positions supported by one or two brief descriptive paragraphs. Because of the importance of the takeoff to the successful execution of springboard dives and the lack of indepth information on this skill, it would seem logical from a biomechanical standpoint to investigate this aspect of the performance and in particular to seek information on the way in which highly skilled female divers generate the required linear momentum and angular momentum for the flight phase of non-twisting springboard dives.

[1] This study was made possible through the cooperation of *Pierre Lagassé* of Laval University and *Kathy Lane* of the Canadian Amateur Diving Association.

Procedure

Films of two female divers on the Canadian National Team were obtained for biomechanical analysis of the springboard takeoff. Subject 1 was 19 years old, with a mess of 62 kg and was 1.43 m in height while subject 2 was 16, (mass 47 kg) and was 1.60 m tall. Both divers were filmed at 100 pps while performing their non-twisting compulsory and optional dives from a 3-m springboard. The compulsories for both divers were the forward dive layout, back dive pike, reverse dive pike and inward dive layout. Both divers performed forward 2½ pike and inward 2½ tuck somersaults as optionals. Optionals from the back and reverse groups were 1½ layout somersaults for subject 1 and 2½ tuck somersaults for subject 2. Each frame ($\Delta t = 0.01$ s) of the takeoffs of these dives was digitized to obtain coordinates of the endpoints of the body segments and the springboard position. These data were smoothed (2nd order Butterworth digital filter with a 4-Hz cutoff) and segmental centers of gravity and angles calculated prior to differentiation to determine relevant velocities and accelerations required in the detailed analysis. Segmental masses, center of gravity locations and moments of inertia were estimated from the data of *Dempster* [1955] and *Chandler* et al. [1975].

Results and Discussion

For the purposes of analysis and reference, the takeoff can be subdivided into two major phases, the depression of the springboard and its subsequent recoil. In forward and reverse dives which have a running approach, these phases are clearly encompassed by the period between the simultaneous two foot landing on the end of the board from the hurdle and the last contact immediately preceding the flight. In backward and inward dives which have a standing approach, the beginning of a comparable takeoff period is more difficult to identify. For consistency, however, it can be taken as the point at which the diver starts the final depression of the springboard. This *follows* initial movements during which the diver raises her arms above her head, balances briefly on the balls of her feet with her ankles plantar-flexed and then accelerates downward by commencing the downswing of the arms in conjunction with hip, knee and ankle flexion. As a consequence of this downward acceleration, the vertical reaction force is less than body weight and the board moves upward. The backward and inward takeoffs then begin as the board starts downward again and, as with the forward and reverse takeoffs, continue until the feet leave the board.

Linear Momentum

The linear momentum which the diver has at the beginning of the takeoff period must be altered by external forces (body weight and springboard re-

action) acting during the takeoff to produce the necessary translation conditions for the flight. By the end of recoil when the diver leaves the board,
she must have sufficient vertical momentum to provide adequate height and
thus enough time in the air to complete the dive as high as possible above the
surface of the water. Further, she must have sufficient horizontal momentum
to take her a safe distance away from the board during the flight but not so
much as to detract from the performance. The way in which skilled divers
change their linear momentum during the takeoff period to accomplish these
objectives is of particular interest. Since linear momentum is the product
of the diver's mass and linear velocity of her center of gravity and, since her
mass remains constant, changes in her momentum are directly reflected by
changes in her velocity.

Vertical. In the present study, downward velocity at the beginning of
the takeoff was almost 1.5 m/s faster for dives with a running approach
(~ -3.4 m/s for forward and reverse) than for those which began from a
standing position (~ -1.9 m/s for backward and inward). On leaving the
board, the upward velocity was approximately 1 m/s higher in dives from
the forward and reverse groups (~ 4.7 and 3.9 m/s for compulsories and
optionals, respectively) than for those from the backward and inward groups
(~ 3.6 and 2.8 m/s for compulsories and optionals, respectively). Further,
across all four groups the upward velocity at the beginning of the flight was
about 1 m/s higher for the compulsory in comparison to the respective
optional dives.

During the entire takeoff period, the diver experiences an upward reaction force from the springboard which, along with body weight, brings
about the changes in vertical velocity just described. The magnitude of the
springboard reaction force depends on: (1) how much kinetic energy was
transferred to the board as a result of the diver's downward velocity at the
beginning of the takeoff; and (2) how much additional force the diver can
superimpose by actively pushing against the board and causing her body to
accelerate upward with respect to the board. This active pushing (or relative
inertia force) is generated by the vertical acceleration of the individual body
segments with respect to the board with each contributing in proportion to
their respective masses ($\sum_{i=1}^{n} m_i (a_i - a_b)$) where a_i is the vertical acceleration of
the segment and a_b is the vertical acceleration of the board.

It has been suggested that the active pushing phase occurs during board
depression and that the diver merely 'rides' the board upward during the

recoil. The results of the present study, however, indicated that although there was a definite active pushing period as the board was depressing, a second active pushing phase was evident toward the end of recoil (fig. 1).

Not surprisingly the trunk accounted for at least half of the upward relative inertia force during springboard depression. Most of its contribution, however, was the result of the legs accelerating the large mass of the trunk upward as the acceleration of the trunk with respect to the hip was small. It was also interesting to note that during this part of board depression the arms and legs made comparable contributions to the upward acceleration of the diver with respect to the board. These forces were associated with the completion of the downswing and beginning of the upswing of the arms and incorporated the eccentric contraction phase of the ankle, knee and hip extensors as the body continued to move downward at the initiation of the takeoff.

During the latter part of recoil when the second active pushing phase was observed, there was a corresponding upward relative inertia force of the legs and also often of the trunk. This may have been associated with extension at the metatarsal-phalangeal joint since the metatarsals were accelerating upward with respect to the board while the accelerations of the feet, lower legs and thighs were small with respect to the metatarsals. In dives from the inward group, this final upward force contribution was almost completely masked by the simultaneous downward acceleration of the trunk with respect to the board (fig. 1).

Horizontal. The horizontal velocity at the beginning of the takeoff for dives with a running approach (i.e. forward and reverse) ranged between 0.6 and 0.8 m/s. In some dives from the backward group a slight 'falling' could be detected as board depression started. Consequently they too had a small amount of horizontal velocity directed away from the board. By contrast, dives from the inward group had zero horizontal velocity at the beginning of takeoff.

In the forward and backward groups, maximum velocity away from the board was reached prior to final contact and decreased slightly before the diver left the board. By contrast, in dives from the reverse and inward groups the highest horizontal velocity coincided with final contact. Although on the average across all dives the velocity at the beginning of the flight was approximately 1 m/s away from the board, dives from the inward group had the smallest and backward optional dives the highest horizontal velocity.

The horizontal component of the springboard reaction force acting

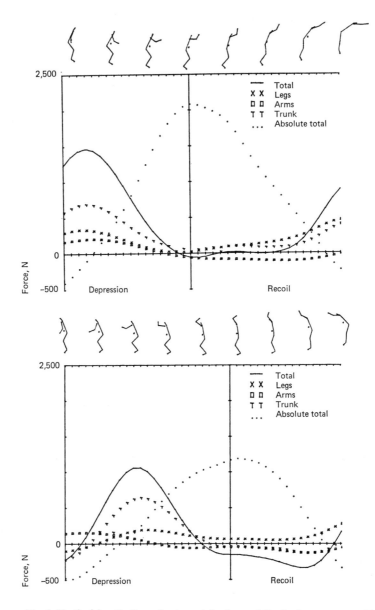

Fig. 1. Vertical inertia force (m*a*) contributions of the body segments with respect to the diving board during the takeoffs for a forward 2½ somersault pike (top) and an inward 2½ somersault tuck (bottom) (subject 2). The total vertical inertia force (i.e. sum of the segment contributions) with respect to the board is shown by the solid line and the ottal vertical inertia force in absolute terms reflecting the vertical acceleration of the diver as a result of her acceleration with respect to the board plus the acceleration of the board is indicated by the dotted line.

upon the diver during depression and the first part of recoil and responsible for the changes in horizontal momentum during this period showed a reasonably consistent pattern for all dives. Following an initial horizontal reaction toward the fulcrum which was small in magnitude and duration and present in most dives, the horizontal reaction was directed toward the tip of the board. Thus, by the middle of the board depression period, the divers had begun to initiate the required impulse to carry them away from the board during the flight (fig. 2).

During the latter part of recoil, the reaction force continued to be directed toward the end of the board in inward and reverse dives and hence the reason for the continuously increasing horizontal velocity. In the forward and backward groups, however, during the terminal portion of the takeoff the horizontal reaction force reduced to near zero in the compulsory dives and was directed toward the fulcrum in the optional dives. Examination of the individual segment inertia forces contributing to this reaction revealed that it was the diver's head and arms which were primarily responsible for this fulcrum directed force in the forward 2½ pike, back 1½ layout (subject 1) and back 2½ tuck (subject 2).

In all four groups of dives the final direction of the horizontal reaction force was consistent with producing rotation in the desired direction for the dive. One can thus understand why unskilled divers sometimes 'cut in' to the board when learning forward and backward somersaults. In their attempt to initiate rotation they rely too much on the moment of the horizontal force and exaggerate the final horizontal impulse toward the fulcrum, reducing their velocity away from the board or perhaps even directing it toward the board with disastrous results!

Angular Momentum

During the takeoff period, the diver must build up sufficient angular momentum to complete the specified number of somersaults during the flight. Once she leaves the board, the only external force influencing her motion is her body weight directed downward through her center of gravity (cg). Since it has no moment or torque about the cg, the total angular momentum with respect to the cg (AM_{cg}) established at the instant the diver leaves the board remains constant.

At the beginning of the takeoff of all dives, there was a small amount of AM_{cg} (~ -2 kg-m^2/s) consistent with forward and backward somersaulting rotation. By the time the diver left the board, the AM_{cg} had increased significantly in magnitude and was in the direction required for rotation of

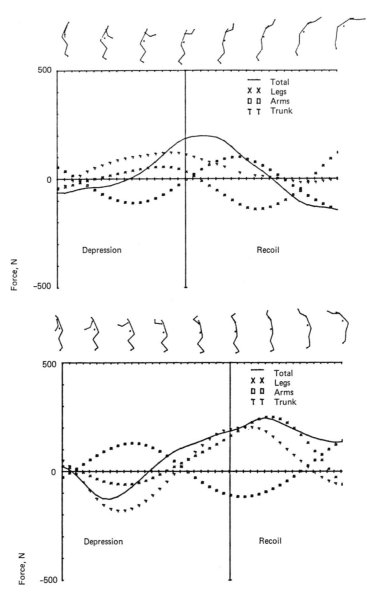

Fig. 2. Horizontal inertia force (ma) contributions of the body segments during the takeoffs for a forward 2½ somersault pike (top) and an inward 2½ somersault tuck (bottom) (subject 2). Positive forces are directed from the fulcrum to the tip of the board and are consistent with the diver's objective to move safely away from the board during the flight. Negative forces act in the opposite direction, toward the fulcrum.

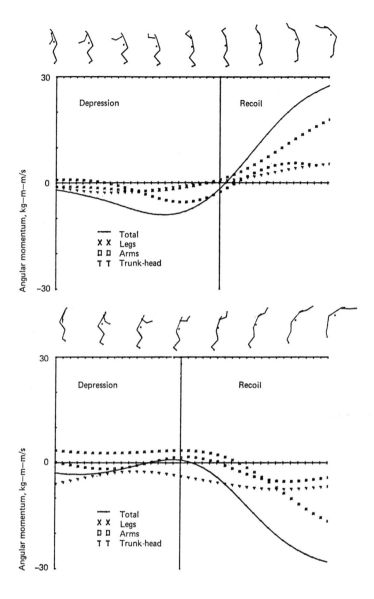

Fig. 3. Angular momentum contributions of the body segments to the total angular momentum with respect to the diver's center of gravity (solid line) during the takeoffs for a forward 2½ somersault pike (bottom) and an inward 2½ tuck (top) (subject 2). The angular momenta shown include both local and remote contributions of the respective segments. Positive angular momentum signifies rotation in a counterclockwise sense which is consistent with the rotation direction required by reverse and inward dives. Negative angular momentum is clockwise and consistent with the rotation direction of dives from forward and backward groups.

the dive being performed. The magnitude of this AM_{cg} was similar for all optional dives of subject 2 ($\sim$ 25–27 kg-m²/s for the forward 2½ pike and back, reverse and inward 2½s tuck) and was 2–3 times greater than for her respective compulsory dives (forward and inward layout and back and reverse pike). The final AM_{cg} for subject 1's back and reverse 1½s layout ($\sim$ 50 kg-m²/s) was noticeably higher than for her forward (pike) and inward (tuck) 2½s (44 and 28 kg-m²/s, respectively).

Analysis of the individual segment contributions to the total AM_{cg} revealed the dominant role of the legs during the final third to half of recoil (fig. 3). This contribution was almost entirely due to the remote AM of the legs (i.e. $r \times mv$ which is the moment of the linear momentum with respect to the cg of the body with r being the position vector joining the body cg to the segment cg, m the segment mass and v the absolute linear velocity of the segment cg) and underlines the importance of the linear velocity of the legs in establishing the required AM_{cg}. For example, if the velocity vector of the legs passes behind the cg in a forward 2½, the remote AM of the legs will promote forward somersaulting rotation. The larger the velocity and the greater the perpendicular distance from the cg to the velocity vector, the greater the remote AM contribution.

Summary

Springboard takeoffs of non-twisting compulsory and optional dives of two female members of the Canadian National Team were analyzed cinematographically. The takeoff was divided into springboard depression and recoil and body segment contributions during these phases were investigated to determine their roles in producing the linear momentum and angular momentum necessary for the flight. The divers appeared to be actively pushing downward against the board not only during depression but also toward the end of recoil. In forward and backward optional dives, the head and arms helped to produce a horizontal reaction force back toward the fulcrum before the divers left the board. In all dives, the remote angular momentum of the legs was found to be the principal contributor to the total angular momentum for the flight.

References

Bergmaier, G.: Biomechanik des Wasserspringens; Diplomarbeit, Zurich (1970).
Bergmaier, G.; Wettstein, A.; Wartenweiler, J.: Diving measurement and analysis of the take-off; in Lewillie, Clarys, Biomechanics in swimming, pp. 243–247 (Université libre de Bruxelles, Brussels 1979).

Chandler, R.F.; Clauser, C.E.; McConville, J.T.; Reynolds, H.M.; Young, J.W.: Investigation of inertial properties of the human body; AMRL-TR-74-137 (Wright-Patterson AFB, Ohio 1975).

Dempster, W.T.: Space requirements of the seated operator; WADC TR 55-159 (Wright-Patterson AFB, Ohio 1955).

Miller, D.I.: A comparative analysis of the take-off employed in springboard dives from the forward and reverse groups; in Nelson, Morehouse, Biomechanics, vol. IV, pp. 223–228 (University Park Press, Baltimore 1974).

Dr. Doris I. Miller, Department of Kinesiology, University of Washington, Seattle, WA 98195 (USA)

Subject Index